SIGHT UNSEEN

SIGHT UNSEEN

An exploration of conscious and unconscious vision

Second Edition

MELVYN GOODALE

DAVID MILNER

OXFORD
UNIVERSITY PRESS

OXFORD
UNIVERSITY PRESS

Great Clarendon Street, Oxford, OX2 6DP,
United Kingdom

Oxford University Press is a department of the University of Oxford.
It furthers the University's objective of excellence in research, scholarship,
and education by publishing worldwide. Oxford is a registered trade mark of
Oxford University Press in the UK and in certain other countries

© Oxford University Press 2013

The moral rights of the authors have been asserted

First Edition published in 2004

Impression: 1

British Library Cataloguing in Publication Data
Data available

ISBN 978–0–19–959696–6

Printed in China by
C & C Offset Printing Co. Ltd.

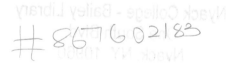

To Deborah, without whom this story could not have been told.

PREFACE

The story of this book began in the early 1970s in St Andrews, Scotland, when the two authors met and first began to work together on research into the workings of the visual system. Our book would not have been written, however, but for the events that unfolded some fifteen years later than that, when the two remarkable people we are calling Dee and Carlo first entered our lives.

By happy coincidence, our first observations on the effects of Dee's brain damage were made at a time when several new developments were emerging in the neuroscience of visually guided movement. This provided fertile soil in which to develop the theoretical notions that we put together in our first book, *The Visual Brain in Action* (Oxford University Press, 1995, 2006). *Sight Unseen*, which was first published in 2004, was an attempt to bring those ideas to a wider audience. In this new edition we have extended and updated *Sight Unseen*, drawing on exciting new findings not only from our own labs, but also from many others. Much of this research has been stimulated by the theoretical ideas that grew out of our early investigations of Dee and her visual world. The new research includes an explosion of work in human brain imaging, as well as in other areas of neuroscience and behavior.

We continue to enjoy the unfailingly cooperative and good-humored help of Dee and Carlo. We are deeply grateful to Dee for sharing her visual world with us and for spending many long hours in the laboratory. We owe them both a deep debt of gratitude. They have taught us not only about the visual brain, but also about how people can overcome the most devastating of problems with fortitude, and still enjoy a rich and happy life. As with all of the brain-damaged patients we describe in the book, Dee's name is fictitious, retaining only her true initials.

We also acknowledge the help at both intellectual and practical levels of many of our colleagues, past and present, especially including (in alphabetical order): Salvatore Aglioti, Stephen Arnott, Jonathan Cant, David Carey, Cristiana Cavina-Pratesi, Craig Chapman, Jason Connolly, Jody Culham, Chris Dijkerman, Richard Dyde, Tzvi Ganel, Richard Gregory, Angela Haffenden, Monika Harvey, Priscilla Heard, David Heeley, Charles Heywood, Yaoping Hu, Keith Humphrey, Lorna

Jakobson, Tom James, Marc Jeannerod, Robert Kentridge, Grzegorz Króliczak, Jonathan Marotta, Robert McIntosh, François Michel, Mark Mon-Williams, Kelly Murphy, David Perrett, Laure Pisella, Nichola Rice-Cohen, Yves Rossetti, Thomas Schenk, Igor Schindler, Philip Servos, Jennifer Steeves, Chris Striemer, Lore Thaler, David Westwood, and Robert Whitwell. We also owe a special thanks to Lynne Mitchell for taking care of all the details associated with arranging Dee's many visits to Canada.

We would also like to thank Gavin Buckingham, Jonathan Cant, Tzvi Ganel, Christine Milner, Paul Milner, Severino Poletto, and Leon Surette for their insightful comments on early drafts of the manuscript—and Kenneth Valyear, Jennifer Steeves, Brian Wandell, Gavin Buckingham, and Rob McIntosh, for their assistance in preparing the figures and illustrations.

CONTENTS

PROLOGUE

Vision, more than any other sense, dominates our mental life. Our visual experience is so rich and detailed that we can hardly distinguish that subjective world from the real thing. Even when we are just thinking about the world with our eyes closed, we can't help imagining what it *looks* like.

But where does that rich visual experience come from? Most of us have the strong impression that we are simply looking out at the world and registering what we see—as if we were nothing more than a rather sophisticated camera that delivers a faithful reproduction of the world on some kind of television screen inside our heads. This idea that we have an internal picture of the world is compelling, yet it turns out to be not only misleading but fundamentally wrong.

There is much more to vision than just pointing our eyes at the world and having the image projected onto an internal screen. Our brain has to make sense of the world, not simply reproduce it. In fact, the brain has to work just as hard to make sense of what's on a television screen in our living room as it does to make sense of the real world itself. So putting the television screen in the brain doesn't explain anything. (Who is looking at the screen in our heads anyway?) But an even more fundamental problem is that our visual *experience* is not all there is to vision. It turns out that some of the most important things that vision does for us never reach our consciousness at all.

One way to get a handle on how vision works is to study what happens when it goes wrong—not just when it goes wrong in the eye but when it goes wrong in the brain. Studying the visual life of people with certain kinds of brain damage has revealed just how misleading our intuitions about how vision works can be. In some cases it is easy to get a feel for what such individuals might experience; in others, as is the case with the woman we are calling "Dee Fletcher" in this book, it can be startlingly difficult to see the world through their eyes.

When we study how brain damage can disturb vision, we do not need to restrict ourselves to wondering how it affects *conscious visual experience*. Of course that is what the brain-damaged person will tell us about. When they talk about their visual problems, they are describing their conscious experience of the world—like the rest of us, they can describe only what they are aware of. But there are other ways of finding out what people can see. If we look at their *behavior* rather than simply listening to what they tell us, we may discover that they have other visual problems not apparent to their own awareness—or in other cases that they may be able to see far more than they think they can.

Trying to understand the visual problems that brain damage can cause leads directly to a more fundamental question: Why do we need vision in the first place? In this book, we take the view that we need vision for two quite different but complementary reasons. On the one hand, we need vision to give us detailed knowledge of the world beyond ourselves—knowledge that allows us to recognize things from minute to minute and day to day. On the other hand, we also need vision to guide our actions in that world at the very moment we are making them. These are two quite different job descriptions, and nature seems to have given us two different visual systems to carry them out. One system, the one that allows us to recognize objects and build up a database about the world, is the one we are more familiar with, the one that gives us our conscious visual experience. The other, much less studied and understood, provides the visual control we need in order to move about and interact with objects. This system does not have to be conscious, but it does have to be quick and accurate.

The idea of two visual systems in a single brain initially seems counterintuitive or even absurd. It seems to conflict with all of our everyday assumptions about how the mind works. In fact, the idea of separate visual systems for perceiving the world and acting on it was not entertained as a plausible scenario even by visual scientists until quite recently. Our visual experience of the world is so compelling that it is hard to believe that a quite separate visual system in the brain, inaccessible to visual consciousness, could be guiding our movements. It seems intuitively obvious that the visual image that allows us to recognize a coffee cup must also guide our hand when we pick it up. But this belief is an illusion. As we try to show in this book, the visual system that gives us our conscious experience of the world is not the visual system that guides our movements in the world.

I

A tragic accident

It was a bright morning in St Andrews, Scotland, in May 1988, when we first heard about Dee Fletcher. We received an unexpected phone call from a colleague at the University of Aberdeen. He had recently returned from Milan where he had heard about a young Scottish woman who had suffered a tragic accident at her new home in Italy. Apparently, the accident had severely affected her sight. She had recently returned to Scotland to stay for a few months with her parents. Would we be interested in examining her? We said we would be happy to help out, although her case did not sound interesting from the point of view of scientific research. Her case looked even less promising when copies of the results of clinical testing carried out in Italy arrived in the mail soon afterwards. Dee had clearly suffered a severe loss of visual function. Her visual problems were not restricted to a single domain such as the ability to recognize faces or to read words—the kind of selective loss that has long held a fascination for psychologists and other scientists interested in how the brain works. Nevertheless, we fixed a date to see her.

A few days later, Dee Fletcher arrived at our St Andrews laboratory. Her mother, who understandably was extremely upset at what had happened to her only daughter, accompanied her. Dee, a small, smartly dressed woman of 34, seemed a bit reserved at first, but soon began to share her unhappy story with us. Dee spoke with the assurance of a well-educated and confident individual, but one who was nevertheless clearly puzzled and distressed about her condition. As she and her mother described her life and how it had been so completely changed by a freak accident, we were able to piece together what had happened.

Dee was born and spent her early years in Scotland, but went on to spend a large part of her life in other countries—including in the Caribbean and in Africa where her father had held a series of university posts. She now lived in Italy, where she had settled down with her partner Carlo, an Italian engineer whom she had met in Nigeria. Dee had completed a college degree in business studies, and this degree, coupled with her fluency in Italian (and several other languages) had enabled her to work as a freelance commercial translator in Italy. She had clearly been an active and lively person with many interests. While in Africa, she had become an accomplished horsewoman and, in the last two years, had learned to fly a private plane. She and her partner had enjoyed a full and happy life. Sadly, one fateful day in February 1988, their life changed forever.

On that day, Dee had been taking a shower in the newly renovated house that she and Carlo had bought in a small village north of Milan. The water for the shower was heated by a propane gas heater—a common practice in many homes in southern Europe at that time. As it turned out, this particular heater was not properly vented and carbon monoxide slowly accumulated in the bathroom. Dee, of course, was unable to detect the fumes, which are quite odorless, and she eventually collapsed into a coma as the carbon monoxide displaced the oxygen in her blood (Box 1.1). There is little doubt she would have died of asphyxiation had Carlo not arrived home just in time to save her. He gave her the kiss of life and rushed her to the local hospital, and she survived. Possibly she would have suffered less brain damage if she could have gained more specialized treatment at that early stage; but at least she survived.

BOX 1.1 CARBON MONOXIDE POISONING

Carbon monoxide (CO) is an invisible odorless gas that is produced whenever fuels such as gasoline, oil, propane, or wood are burned. Dangerous amounts of CO can accumulate when fuel-burning appliances are not properly vented. CO poisoning occurs because CO displaces blood-borne oxygen (by competing successfully with the oxygen molecule for sites on the hemoglobin molecule). The most common symptoms of CO poisoning are headache, dizziness, weakness, nausea, vomiting, chest pain, and confusion. High levels of carbon monoxide can cause loss of consciousness and death. In fact, CO is the number-one cause of unintentional poisoning deaths in the world. The main way CO kills is by depriving the brain of oxygen. In other words, CO poisoning causes anoxia.

Anoxia is a condition in which there is an absence of oxygen supply to an organ's tissues even though there is adequate blood flow to the organ. Hypoxia is a milder form of anoxia. The brain is particularly sensitive to the loss of oxygen and brain cells cannot function without oxygen for more than a few minutes.

The vast majority of people who survive carbon monoxide poisoning show few, if any, noticeable neurological effects. It was obvious to Carlo, however, as soon as Dee regained consciousness, that she was not among that fortunate majority, and he feared the worst. While she seemed alert and could speak and understand what was said to her, she could see nothing. The initial diagnosis of local doctors was therefore "cortical blindness." This is a condition caused by damage to the primary visual area at the back of the brain, depriving the individual of all visual experience. But gradually in the days following her arrival at the hospital, Dee began to regain some conscious sight. The first visual experience that she recalls having is a vivid sensation of color. Dee could see the red and green colors of the flowers in the vase beside her bed and the blue and white of the sky outside. She remarked to Carlo that he was wearing the same blue sweater he had worn the day before. It was now clear that Dee did not have cortical blindness.

Nevertheless, Mrs Fletcher, who had flown out to Italy to be with her daughter, was devastated when she walked into the hospital room and Dee looked at her but did not recognize who she was. Dee immediately recognized her voice, however, and Mrs Fletcher was relieved to discover as she talked to her daughter that Dee could still remember everyday things and talk about them in her usual way. She realized that while Dee's problems were serious, they seemed to be largely restricted to seeing things properly and making sense of them. For example, Dee had no trouble telling what things were when she picked them up and explored them by touch.

The following day, Dee and her mother talked together over coffee. As Mrs Fletcher passed a cup to her daughter, Dee said something rather startling: "You know what's peculiar, Mum? I can see the tiny hairs on the back of your hand!" This surprising remark led her mother to think that perhaps Dee's sight was on the road to a full recovery. But her hopes were dashed when Dee added that, despite seeing those fine details, she could not make out the shape of her mother's hand as a whole. In fact it soon became apparent that Dee was completely lost when it came to the shape and form of things around her. Unless an object had a distinctive color, visual texture, or surface detail she had no idea what it was. And over the next few days and weeks it became painfully clear to all concerned that Dee's vision was no longer improving.

Vision without shape

As we heard this story, it became apparent to us that Dee's visual problems could not be due to a general deterioration in her visual system. For one thing, even though she could not use shape to tell one object from another, she could still use their surface detail and color. This ability to see surface properties was confirmed in formal

3

testing that we later carried out with Dee in St Andrews. We found that she could not only name colors correctly but was also able to make fine discriminations between different shades of the same color. She could also distinguish the surface features of many objects, allowing her to identify the material they were made from (see Figure 1.1, torch). So she might say that an object was made of red plastic or out of shiny metal—while at the same time she could only guess at its shape or function. In some cases, of course, color and other surface features can be highly diagnostic of what kind of object a picture represents (like the yellow color of a banana or the tiny seeds on the surface of a strawberry; see Figure 1.2 for another example).

We tested Dee's ability to see fine detail (like the hairs on her mother's hand and the seeds on a strawberry) formally, by showing her patterns of lines on a computer screen. She did as well as a normally-sighted person in detecting a circular "Gabor" patch of closely spaced fine lines on a background that had the same average brightness (see Figure 1.3). Yet, remarkably, even though she could see that there was a patch of lines there, Dee was completely unable to say whether the lines were horizontal or vertical. Of course, the fact that she could see detail just as well as a person with normal sight ruled out one obvious explanation of the problem she had in recognizing the shapes of objects. That is, it could not be the case that her vision was simply a blur—as it would be for a short-sighted person without their eye glasses. Dee, unlike the person with myopia, *could* see the detail. It was the edges and outlines of objects that she couldn't make out. Her difficulty in telling even horizontal from vertical lines shows just how extreme this deficit was.

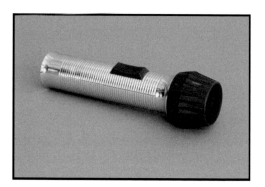

Figure 1.1 When this cheap flashlight was placed on the table in front of Dee, she said: "It's made of aluminium. It's got red plastic on it. Is it some sort of kitchen utensil?" She guessed it was something for the kitchen—probably because a lot of kitchen implements are made of metal and plastic. As soon as the flashlight was placed in her hand, Dee knew exactly what it was. "Oh. It's an electric torch!" she said.

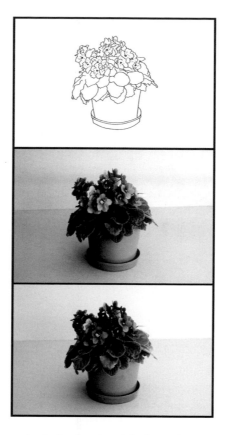

Figure 1.2 Dee cannot recognize the line drawing of the flower shown here. Nor does she do much better with a black and white photograph. Dee can recognize objects depicted in color photographs, however—particularly if the color and other surface features are "diagnostic" of the object. When presented with the color photograph shown here, for example, she said "Oh! It's a flower. I think it's an African violet." She doesn't use the color-defined edges to see the shape of an object; instead she appears to use color to identify its material properties. In other words, she sees the textures and colors of the leaves and petals of the African violet without seeing its overall shape.

Dee has never regained a full and integrated experience of the visual world. The world she sees still lacks shape and form. So even today, more than twenty years after the accident, Dee remains unable to identify objects on the basis of their form alone. She has never, for example, been able to recognize printed letters or digits on paper, or the faces of her friends and relatives, nor drawings or photographs of everyday objects. She has great difficulty in following a program or movie on television, especially one in black and white or in cartoon form, though she enjoys listening to audio CDs of novels, read by an actor or the author, intended for the visually impaired.

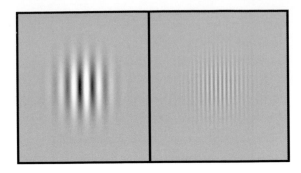

Figure 1.3 Examples of the several Gabor "grating" patterns used to test Dee's vision for fine detail. (These patches were first devised by Dennis Gabor, a Nobel laureate in Physics, who is most famous for working out the theory behind holograms.) The number of stripes per unit distance is called the spatial frequency of the pattern—the grating on the left has a low spatial frequency, the one on the right has a high spatial frequency. For each pattern, we determined the degree of contrast between dark and light stripes that was needed for Dee to see it reliably against a gray background with the same overall brightness. Dee did remarkably well in detecting these faint patterns, especially at the high spatial frequencies, even though she could not reliably tell us whether the stripes were horizontal, vertical, or diagonal.

We discovered early on that Dee even had problems in separating an object from its background—sometimes called "figure-ground segregation"—a basic first step for the brain in working out what an object is. Dee said that objects seemed to "run into each other," so that two adjacent objects of a similar color, such as a knife and fork, will often look to her like a single entity. Conversely, she will sometimes see two differently colored parts of a single object as two different objects.

It was very apparent that Dee had difficulty naming even the simplest geometrical shapes, like a triangle, a square, an oblong, or a diamond. We began by showing her line drawings of shapes, or filled-in black shapes on a white background. But she was no better when we showed her shapes that differed from their backgrounds in color instead of brightness. In other words, although she could see the colors all right, she couldn't make out the edges between them. Neither could she recognize a shape made up of random dots set against a background with a different density of dots. Nor could she see "shape from motion" where a patch of dots is moved against a background of similar but stationary dots. A person with normal vision will see the shape immediately (though it soon fades, rather like Lewis Carroll's Cheshire Cat, once the motion has stopped). Dee saw *something* moving under these circumstances, and could tell us in which direction—but she was quite unable to tell us what the shape was. To cut a long story short, it did not matter how a shape was

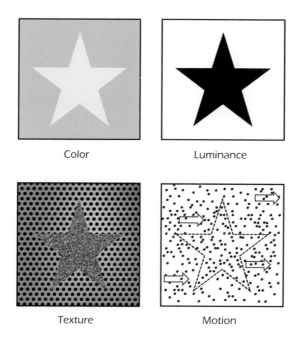

Figure 1.4 The edges of objects can be defined in a number of different ways. They can be defined by differences in luminance (a boundary between light and dark regions), differences in color, differences in visual texture, or differences in the direction of motion. In everyday life, the edges or boundaries of objects are typically determined by combinations of these different cues. Thus, when we see a dark green van driving down a snowy road, differences in luminance, color, visual texture, and motion all contribute to our perception of the van. When shown the patterns depicted here, Dee could not make out the star shape in any of them.

defined, whether by brightness, color, texture, or motion, Dee still could not recognize it (see Figure 1.4).

Dee's difficulty in identifying objects or line drawings is not one of finding the right name for the object, nor is it one of knowing or remembering what common objects look like. Her problem is more fundamentally "visual" than that. For example, Dee has great difficulties in copying drawings of common objects or geometric shapes (see Figure 1.5). Some brain-damaged patients who are unable to identify pictures of objects can still slavishly copy what they see, line by line, and produce something recognizable. But Dee can't even pick out the individual edges and contours that make up a picture in order to copy them. Presumably, unlike those other patients, Dee's problem is not one of *interpreting* a picture that she sees clearly—her problem is that she can't see the shapes in the picture to start with.

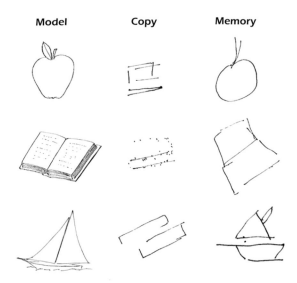

Figure 1.5 Dee was unable to recognize any of the drawings in the left-hand column. In fact, as the middle column shows, she could not even make recognizable copies of the drawings. When she tried to copy the book, Dee did incorporate some of the elements from the original drawing—the small dots representing text, for example—but her copy as a whole was unrecognizable. After all, she had no idea what she was copying. Dee's inability to copy the drawings was not due to a failure to control her finger and hand movements as she moved the pencil on the paper, since on another occasion, when asked to draw (for example) an apple from memory, she produced reasonable renditions, as shown in the right-hand column. Dee was presumably able to do this because she still has memories of what objects like apples look like. Yet when she was later shown her own drawings from memory, she had no idea what they were. Reproduced from Milner, A.D. and Goodale, M.A. *Visual Brain in Action*, Figure 5.2 © 1995, Oxford University Press, with permission.

Yet despite her copying problems, Dee can draw pictures of many common objects from memory. For example, when asked to "draw an apple" or "draw a house," she does this quite well (see Figure 1.5). Her drawings are by no means perfect, but then it is almost as if she is drawing with her eyes closed, because she does not appreciate visually what she is drawing. It is not surprising that sometimes the parts of the drawing are misaligned, because when she lifts the pencil from the page she does not always put it back again in the right place (Figure 1.6). But the fact that she draws from memory as well as she does means that her problem with copying drawings is not that she can no longer draw, nor is it that she has lost her general knowledge of what objects look like.

When Dee is "drawing from memory" she can rely on visual experiences she had before her accident. It seems that Dee has as rich a store of visual memories and

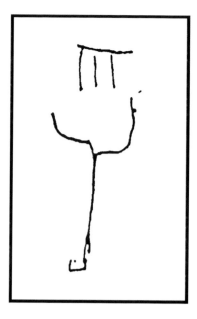

Figure 1.6 As shown in Figure 1.5, Dee can draw quite well from memory even though later she can't recognize what she has drawn. Indeed, she can't see what she is drawing even when she's actually moving her pencil on the page. Thus, when she tries to draw a multi-part object like a fork, she is liable to lose track of where she left off and as a consequence continue her drawing in the wrong place, as in this example. Reproduced from Goodale, M.A. The cortical organization of visual perception and visuomotor control. In S. Kosslyn (ed.), *An Invitation to Cognitive Science. Vol. 2. Visual Cognition and Action* (2nd edition), Figure 5.2 © MIT Press, 1995, with permission.

visual knowledge as anyone else—apart from the fact that these memories have not been updated with new visual information during the years since her accident (although of course she would still be constantly reminded of the shapes of small everyday objects through her sense of touch, from handling them now and then). But unfortunately Dee's ability to draw from memory does not help her deal with new visual information—indeed she recognizes her own drawings no better than she recognizes drawings by others.

Her general knowledge about the appearance of objects enables Dee to bring visual images of familiar things into consciousness and talk and think about them. The ability to see things "in our mind's eye" allows us to carry out mental operations on objects when the objects are not actually present. Suppose you are asked to say whether a particular animal has a tail that is longer than its body. You will probably do this by conjuring up a visual image of the animal. Examining this image allows you to say that a mouse, for example, has a tail longer than its body, while a cow does not. Dee can do this just as well as most people, and readily comes up with the right answers. She can even do things involving quite complex mental operations. Take the following case: "Think of the capital letter D; now imagine that it has been rotated flat-side down; now put it on top of the capital letter V; what does it look like?" Most people will say "an ice-cream cone"—and so does Dee.

So Dee can imagine things that her brain damage prevents her from seeing. After all, she is completely unable to recognize an actual letter D or V when she sees one. This must mean that manipulating images in the mind's eye does not depend on exactly the same parts of the brain that allow us to see things out there in the world. Indeed, if visual imagination did depend on those brain structures, then Dee should not have been able to imagine things at all—at least visually.

Not only can Dee deliberately form mental images, but she also finds herself doing so involuntarily at night when dreaming. She still sometimes reports experiencing a full visual world in her dreams, as rich in people, objects, and scenes as her dreams used to be before the accident. Waking up from dreams like this, especially in the early years, was a depressing experience for her. Remembering her dream as she gazed around the bedroom, she was cruelly reminded of the visual world she had lost.

Visual agnosia

Dee's basic problem is in recognizing shapes. In cases such as hers, where brain damage causes a disturbance in people's ability to recognize things, the disorder is known as "agnosia." This term was coined in the late 19th century by a then little-known neurologist named Sigmund Freud. He borrowed two elements from the ancient Greek (*a* = not, and *gnosis* = knowledge), in order to capture the idea that patients of this kind have a problem in understanding what they see. Although we are focusing here on visual deficits, agnosias can be found in other senses, such as touch and hearing. Within vision itself, agnosia can be limited to particular visual categories, such as faces, places, or even words.

Even before Freud wrote about it, a distinction had been made by the German neurologist Heinrich Lissauer between two forms of agnosia (which at that earlier time was called "mind-blindness" or *Seelenblindheit*). According to Lissauer, agnosia could be caused by a disconnection either between perception and meaning, on the one hand, or between sensation and perception on the other (see Figure 1.7). The influential Massachusetts Institute of Technology (MIT) neuroscientist Hans-Lukas Teuber characterized the first of these disorders (what is generally called "associative" agnosia) as one that left people with "percepts stripped of their meaning." In other words, although their visual experience was intact, patients with associative

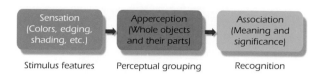

Stimulus features   Perceptual grouping   Recognition

Figure 1.7 During the 19th century, the prevailing view was that we put together our raw sensations into percepts, and then attach associations to these to give them significance. Heinrich Lissauer believed that either of these two links could be severed to cause a brain-damaged person to lose the ability to recognize what he or she saw. If the first link was broken, then the person would have "apperceptive agnosia," while if the second was broken he or she would have "associative agnosia." We retain broadly the same ideas today, though the terminology is different.

agnosia could no longer attach meaning to that experience. To imagine what this would be like, think about what a typical Westerner experiences when faced with a Chinese ideogram. This symbol—full of meaning for a Chinese speaker—would be perfectly well perceived, but nonetheless remain a meaningless and puzzling pattern for the Westerner. A patient with associative agnosia would presumably react in the same uncomprehending way when faced with a drawing of a common object such as a telephone or a bicycle. They would be able to copy the picture quite accurately (as we could do with an ideogram), but they would not have the slightest inkling of what it was they were drawing.

The other kind of agnosia that Lissauer described, which he conceptualized as a disconnection between sensation and perception, is generally called "apperceptive" agnosia. In making this distinction between sensation and perception, Lissauer was using psychological concepts that were fashionable at the time. For the 19th-century thinker, sensation meant the raw sensory qualities like the color, motion, and brightness of objects or their parts, while perception referred to the process that put all of these elements together to create our visual experience, or "percept," of an object, such as a table or a tree. A patient with apperceptive agnosia, then, would not perceive the world properly, though he or she might have perfectly intact sensory data. Because their brains cannot reconstruct the world from the information their eyes provide, they would be unable to copy line drawings of tables, trees, or even simple geometric shapes.

Nowadays, Lissauer's rationale for the distinctions he was making is regarded as a little simplistic. He perhaps put too much emphasis on what today would be called "bottom-up" processing, in which the percept is constructed directly from an analysis of the pattern of light falling on the eye. Today, most visual scientists believe that such bottom-up processing, while certainly necessary, is far from sufficient for perception. They argue that what we see is also shaped by what we *know* about the

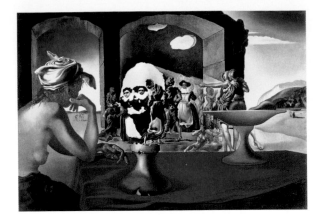

Figure 1.8 Detail from *Slave Market with the Disappearing Bust of Voltaire*. Salvador Dali was an expert at devising paintings in which more than one image is depicted. Top-down knowledge about the shapes of faces causes one to see the bust of Voltaire, in which the facial features are actually made up of two female figures dressed in black and white clothing. Alternatively, one can choose to see the figures rather than Voltaire. © Salvador Dali, Fundació Gala-Salvador Dali, DACS, 2012.

world: in other words that learning, memory, and expectations play a crucial role in molding our perceptions. The contribution of these influences from the brain's knowledge-base about the world is often referred to as "top-down" processing. The final percept is based on a dynamic interaction between the current sensory input and stored information from past experience (see Figure 1.8).

Despite these reservations, most clinicians would agree that Lissauer's classification scheme still provides a useful rule of thumb for distinguishing between different levels of agnosia. Dee, of course, would fall into Lissauer's "apperceptive" category. Her percepts are far from normal, and she certainly cannot produce recognizable copies of line drawings. So Dee's problems correspond well with Lissauer's conception of apperceptive agnosia. But since Lissauer's time, the designation "apperceptive agnosia" has been used by different writers to refer to a range of different perceptual problems, not all of which involve such a basic disorder of shape perception. To avoid confusion, therefore, we will avoid using that particular term. Instead, we will follow the neurologists Frank Benson and John Greenberg of Boston University, who in 1969 coined the more suitably descriptive term "visual form agnosia" for a famous patient of theirs whose basic problem, like Dee's, lay in perceiving visual form or shape. In fact, their patient, who was systematically studied by the American psychologist Robert Efron in a seminal paper published in 1969, was uncannily similar to Dee Fletcher in a number of ways. "Mr S." (as Efron referred to him) had suffered a carbon monoxide poisoning accident while taking a shower, just like Dee

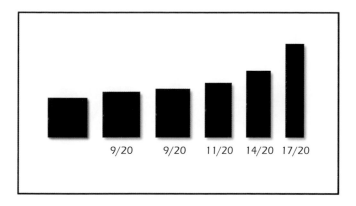

9/20   9/20   11/20   14/20   17/20

Figure 1.9 Efron's rectangles: these all have the same surface area but differ in shape. Dee was tested with several different rectangles, each in a separate test run. On each test trial, she was shown a pair of shapes, either two squares, two rectangles, or one of each (with the square either on the right or the left). She was asked to say whether the two shapes were the same or different. When we used any of the three rectangles that were most similar to the square, she performed at chance level. She sometimes even made mistakes when we used the most elongated rectangle, despite taking a long time to decide. Under each rectangle is the number of correct judgments (out of 20) that Dee made in a test run with that particular rectangle.

did twenty years later. And like Dee, he was able to distinguish colors, but was quite unable to distinguish among geometric shapes.

Efron devised what is now a standard diagnostic test of visual form agnosia (see Figure 1.9). In order to measure the degree of disability a patient had in distinguishing shapes, Efron needed a test where the level of difficulty could be scaled, so that the degree of deficit in different patients could be graded. He hit upon the idea of creating a series of rectangular shapes that varied in length and width but not in area. These objects could be distinguished only by attending to their relative dimensions, not to their overall size. We have tested Dee using these shapes on a number of different occasions over the years. She still has great difficulty in telling pairs of these "Efron shapes" apart, and even when she gets them right, she seems to arrive at her answer through a long and arduous process far removed from the immediacy of normal visual perception.

When we first began working with Dee, we did not have access to the high-resolution brain scanners that are nowadays commonplace in hospitals in the developed world. However, during her initial hospitalization in Italy, Dee was given a preliminary computed tomography scan, which gave us a rough idea of where the damage was that caused her visual problems (see Box 1.2 for terms describing the brain's geography). As shown in Figure 1.10, the "cerebral hemispheres," which dominate the brain

13

BOX 1.2 DESCRIBING THE BRAIN'S GEOGRAPHY

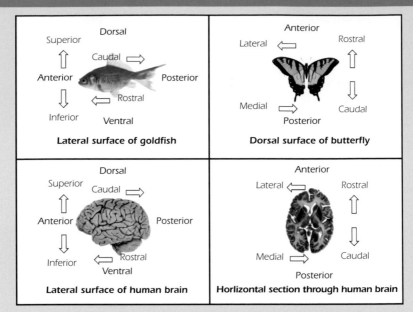

Lateral surface of goldfish	**Dorsal surface of butterfly**
Lateral surface of human brain	**Horlizontal section through human brain**

There are standard conventions for referring to directions and locations within the nervous system. In fact, these same terms are used to describe the relations between parts of the body in all organisms. Some of the terms reflect the names of actual body parts themselves. Thus, the terms *rostral* and *caudal* are derived from the Latin for head and tail respectively—and the terms *dorsal* and *ventral* also come from Latin words, in this case for the back and the belly. Although the origin of these terms makes perfect sense in creatures like the fish and the butterfly, things are not quite so literal in the case of the human brain and the brains of other higher primates that have an upright posture. In fact, unlike most mammals we are so thoroughly bipedal that our brain is turned 90° forward with respect to the long axis of our body (and our spinal cord). Nevertheless, the same "geographical" terms are still used because they allow meaningful comparisons to be made between our brains and the brains of other species. The other terms are fairly self-explanatory: medial means towards the midline, lateral towards the side.

in humans, are conventionally divided into "lobes," whose names are derived from the cranial bones that weld together during infancy to form the skull. The occipital lobe lies at the back of the brain, and it was here that the most conspicuous damage in Dee's brain was found, extending around the junction between the occipital and temporal lobes on the lateral sides of the two hemispheres. Her accident, however, did not destroy the very backmost part of the occipital lobe, where the visual information

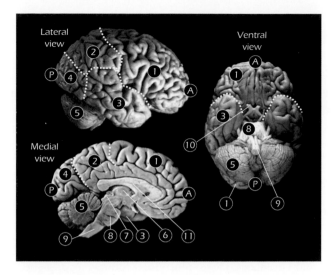

Figure 1.10 The human brain, showing the lateral, medial, and ventral surfaces.
Key: A, anterior; P, posterior; 1, frontal lobe; 2, parietal lobe; 3, temporal lobe; 4, occipital lobe; 5, cerebellum; 6, thalamus; 7, superior colliculus; 8, pons; 9, medulla; 10, optic nerve; 11, corpus callosum.

first arrives at the two hemispheres. This would fit with the fact that Dee was not completely bereft of any visual experience. As we shall see in later chapters, the location of her damage close to the occipito-temporal junction was highly significant.

Summary

After three sessions of testing in our St Andrews laboratory, it was obvious to us that Dee had a profound visual form agnosia. At the same time, her memory, her ability to express herself verbally, and her senses of hearing and touch were all remarkably unaffected by the asphyxia that had devastated her visual experience of the world. And even here the damage was selective, with only some aspects of visual experience being affected. Her experience of color and the surface "texture" of objects seemed to be relatively normal. In other words, Dee's visual form agnosia appeared to be an unusually pure one. It was also obvious to us from the moment she walked into our laboratory that Dee did not suffer from any serious motor disability. That is, she had no problems walking or using her hands to pick things up. In fact, all her motor abilities seemed normal—which is often not the case in other patients who have survived near-asphyxiation. As we shall see in Chapter 2, this sparing of Dee's motor system turned out to be highly significant for our further investigations.

15

Further Reading

An English translation of Lissauer's classic paper on visual agnosia is provided by:

Shallice, T. and Jackson, M. (1988). Lissauer on agnosia. *Cognitive Neuropsychology*, 5, 153–192. (Translation of: Lissauer, H. (1890). [A case of visual agnosia with a contribution to theory.] *Archiv für Psychiatrie*, 21, 222–270.)

For an authoritative review of the varieties of visual agnosias, see:

Farah, M.J. (2004). *Visual Agnosia* (2nd edition). Cambridge, MA: MIT Press/Bradford Books.

There are two classic papers on Mr S., a patient who also experienced a hypoxic episode from carbon monoxide inhalation, and whose resulting deficits were remarkably similar to Dee's:

Benson, D.F. and Greenberg, J.P. (1969). Visual form agnosia: a specific deficit in visual discrimination. *Archives of Neurology 20*, 82–89.

Efron, R. (1969). What is perception? *Boston Studies in the Philosophy of Science*, 4, 137–173.

For an overview of other cases like Dee and Mr S. that have been reported in the literature, see the following review:

Heider, B. (2000). Visual form agnosia: neural mechanisms and anatomical foundations. *Neurocase*, 6, 1–12.

The following book gives an interesting account of the different types of agnosia, along with a detailed description of a particular case, John, who has a different form of the disorder from Dee:

Humphreys, G.W. and Riddoch M.J. (2013). *To See But Not to See: A case study of visual agnosia*. Hove: Psychology Press.

II

Doing without seeing

The picture painted in Chapter 1 is a gloomy one. Dee's brain damage left her with a profoundly diminished visual life. Not only is she unable to recognize her friends and relatives, she cannot even tell the difference between simple shapes like squares and rectangles or triangles and circles. Indeed, a task as straightforward as distinguishing between horizontal and vertical lines defeats her. Given such a profound disability, the prognosis when we first met Dee was discouraging. Most clinicians would have classified her as legally blind, relegating her to a life in which she would need a white cane—or even a guide dog—in order to move about. After all, she could not identify anything on the basis of its shape or form. How could she possibly be expected to use her eyes to do even simple everyday tasks, such as eating a meal? Of course, many blind people can manage such tasks quite well by non-visual means. But would she, like a blind person, have to rely entirely on memory and the sense of touch?

This scenario, happily enough, has not materialized. Quite remarkably, Dee behaves in many everyday situations as though she sees perfectly well. We caught our first glimpse of Dee's preserved visual skills during one of the early testing sessions in St Andrews, back in the summer of 1988. At that time, we were showing her various everyday objects to see whether she could recognize them, without allowing her to feel what they were. When we held up a pencil, we were not surprised that she couldn't tell us what it was, even though she could tell us it was yellow. In fact, she had no idea whether we were holding it horizontally or vertically. But then something quite extraordinary happened. Before we knew it, Dee had reached out

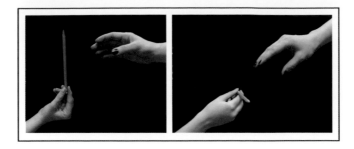

Figure 2.1 The examiner held a pencil either vertically (left picture) or horizontally (right). Even though Dee had no idea whether the pencil was vertical or horizontal, she always grasped it perfectly.

and taken the pencil, presumably to examine it more closely (see Figure 2.1). After a few moments, it dawned on us what an amazing event we had just witnessed. By performing this simple everyday act she had revealed a side to her vision which, until that moment, we had never suspected was there. Dee's movements had been quick and perfectly coordinated, showing none of the clumsiness or fumbling that one might have expected in someone whose vision was as poor as hers. To have grasped the pencil in this skillful way, she must have turned her wrist "in flight" so that her fingers and thumb were well positioned in readiness for grasping the pencil—just like a fully sighted person. Yet it was no fluke: when we took the pencil back and asked her to do it again, she always grabbed it perfectly, no matter whether we held the pencil horizontally, vertically, or obliquely.

Dee's ability to perform this simple act presented a real paradox. How could she see the location, orientation, and shape of the pencil well enough to posture her hand correctly as she reached out to grasp it, while at the same time she couldn't tell us what she saw? She certainly could not have grasped the pencil accurately *without* using vision. A blind person couldn't have done it, nor could a sighted person wearing a blindfold. For her to have grasped the pencil so deftly, her brain must have had all kinds of advance information about where it was and what it looked like. Since there was no other way she could know how we were holding the pencil, Dee had to be using vision. Yet at the same time it was clear that she wasn't using conscious vision. It was this serendipitous observation that first made us suspect that Dee had visual abilities that even she was not aware of—abilities that had survived her loss of conscious visual experience.

Once we had realized what had happened, we began to notice new examples of Dee's amazing visual abilities every time we met with her. The contrast between what she could *perceive* and what she could actually *do* with her sense of vision could not have struck us more forcibly than it did one day when a group of us went out on a picnic while visiting her in Italy. We had spent the morning at her home carrying out a series of visual tests, recording one failure after another. Dee was unable to recognize any of the faces, patterns, or drawings we showed to her. Again it was obvious that the only way Dee could even tell one person from another was by looking at the color of their hair or their clothing. It had been a frustrating morning for her.

To lighten the gloom, Carlo suggested that we all go for a picnic in the Italian Alps, to a popular spot not far from their home. We drove high up into the mountains, until the massive peak of Monrosa loomed into view. We parked the car and then set off on foot to reach our picnic site—an alpine meadow higher up on the side of the mountain. This walk provided a good example of a time when the other side of Dee's visual life was strikingly revealed. To reach the meadow, we had to walk along a half-mile trail through a dense pine forest. The footpath was steep and uneven. Yet Dee had no trouble at all. She walked confidently and unhesitatingly, without stumbling, tripping over a root, or colliding with the branches of the trees that hung over the path. Occasionally we had to point out to her the correct route to take, but other than that, her behavior was indistinguishable from that of any of the other hikers on the mountain that day.

We eventually arrived at the meadow and began to unpack the picnic hamper. Here Dee displayed once more how apparently normal her visual behavior was. She reached out to take things that were passed to her with the same confidence and skill as someone with completely normal sight. No one would ever have guessed that she could not see the difference between a knife and a fork, or recognize the faces of her companions.

The mailbox

Needless to say, scientific colleagues are seldom convinced by anecdotes like these, however compelling they might seem at the time. We had to demonstrate Dee's visual skills in the laboratory. We had to show that even though she was unable to recognize objects or even tell them apart, this did not prevent her from using vision to guide her actions directed at those objects. And this meant introducing both objective measurement and experimental control. Our first attempt to do this was inspired by that remarkable day when she reached out and grasped a pencil during our preliminary tests of object recognition. Refining a test first described by Marie-Thérèse Perenin and Alain Vighetto (see Chapter 3), we set up a simple piece of apparatus where we could ask Dee to "post" a card into an open slot—like a mailbox, but with the added feature that the slot could be presented at different orientations, not just at the horizontal (see Figure 2.2). On each occasion, she had

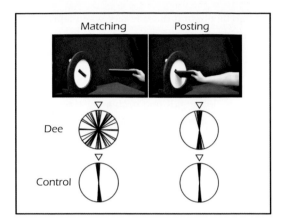

Figure 2.2 Matching and posting tasks. Dee was presented with a vertical display with a slot cut into it which could be rotated to different orientations. In the "matching" task, she was asked to turn a hand-held card so that it matched with the orientation of the slot, without reaching out toward the display. In the "posting" task, she was asked to reach out and "post" the card into the slot. As shown in the diagrams below the pictures, Dee had no problem with the posting task, but performed almost randomly on the matching task. Healthy control subjects, of course, had no problem with either task. (Although the slot was presented in several different orientations, the diagrams show "correct" as vertical.) Reproduced from Goodale, M.A., Milner, A.D., Jakobson, L.S., & Carey, D.P., A neurological dissociation between perceiving objects and grasping them. *Nature, 349,* pp. 154–156 (Figure 1) © 1991, Nature Publishing Group, with permission.

no way of knowing ahead of time what the orientation of the slot would be when she opened her eyes to look at it.

When tested in this way, Dee performed remarkably well, whatever the orientation of the slot. Indeed the accuracy of her behavior was almost indistinguishable from that of several people with unimpaired vision that we tested. Dee moved her hand forward unhesitatingly, and almost always inserted the card smoothly into the slot. Moreover, video recordings revealed that she began to rotate the card toward the correct orientation well in advance of arriving at the slot. In other words, she was using vision right from the start of each movement—just as anyone with normal vision would do. Over the years, we have tested her on several versions of this test and her behavior always looks normal, however we measure it.

Given what we knew about Dee's visual abilities, we were pretty sure that she wouldn't be able to tell us about the different orientations of the slot—even though she was inserting the card into it so accurately. But we had to check this formally. In our first attempt to do this, we simply asked her to tell us what the orientation of the slot was—was it horizontal, vertical, or tilted to the left or right? Most of the time she appeared to have little idea of the slot's orientation and ended up simply guessing. For example, she was just as likely to say that a vertical slot was horizontal as she was to get it right. But this was still not convincing enough—maybe her problem was not so much a visual one but rather one of putting what she saw into words. So in another test, we asked her to tell us the orientation by simply lifting the card up and turning it to match the orientation of the slot, but without making a reaching movement towards the slot. Here we were not asking her to use words to tell us what she saw, but to use her hand to *show* us what she saw. But the videotapes we made of her hand rotations told much the same story as her verbal descriptions. In other words, the angles at which she held the card showed no relationship at all to the actual orientation of the slot.

Her failure to "match" the slot correctly using the card was not simply because she couldn't rotate her hand properly to indicate an orientation she had in mind. We were able to rule out that possibility by asking her to *imagine* a slot at different orientations. Once she had done this, she had no difficulty rotating the card to show us the orientation she'd been asked to imagine. It was only when she had to look at a real slot and match its orientation that her deficit appeared.

These first experimental tests confirmed our suspicions that something very interesting was going on. Dee could turn her hand correctly so that the card would pass smoothly into the slot, but she could not make a similar rotation of her hand to convey to us the orientation of the slot that she saw in front of her. But this was just the beginning of the story.

Grasping size

The posting test showed that Dee had good visual control of her hand movements when confronted with an oriented slot. Of course whenever we pick up a pencil we unthinkingly tailor the orientation of our hand to the orientation of the pencil. At the same time, we also calibrate the separation of our finger and thumb as we move our hand toward the pencil. We do all this quite automatically. In fact, our hand and fingers begin to adopt the final posture of the grasp well before we make contact. In doing this, the advance information we use has to be visual—particularly when we are confronted with the object for the first time and so we have no memory of it to fall back on.

The exquisite tuning of the hand to the target of the grasp was first documented in detail by the late French neuroscientist Marc Jeannerod. He made high-speed films of normal individuals reaching out to grasp solid objects like balls and cylinders of different sizes. By then looking at individual frames of film, he was able to reconstruct the entire trajectory of the grasping movement from start to finish. These reconstructions revealed a beautifully orchestrated action. As soon as the hand left the table en route to the object, the fingers and thumb began to open (see Figure 2.3). Then, about

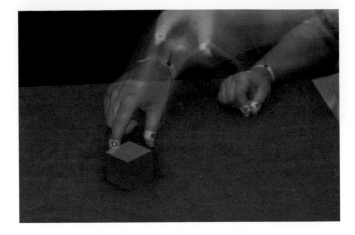

Figure 2.3 This sequence shows a hand reaching out to grasp a wooden block. Notice that the finger and thumb first open wider than the block and then close down as the hand approaches the block. The maximum extent of opening is referred to as the "maximum grip aperture," or MGA.

three-quarters of the way toward the object, they began to close in on the object so that a smooth and accurate grasp was achieved. Even though the maximum opening between the fingers and thumb was much larger than the width of the object itself, Jeannerod showed that the two were closely related: the bigger the object, the bigger the maximum grip size (see Figure 2.4 and Box 2.1).

So the obvious next question to ask was this: Would Dee show the same relationship between grip size and object size that Jeannerod had demonstrated in healthy people—even though she had no conscious visual experience of the dimensions of the objects?

We already knew that she had no difficulty picking up everyday objects of many different shapes and sizes, from pencils to coffee cups. But to test this more formally, we had to come up with some objects where the dimensions could be varied but the overall size of the object did not change. Also, it was important to use objects that had no meaning, so that she couldn't simply remember what kind of grasp was required by guessing what the object was. For example, she might guess that she was picking up a pencil from its yellow color, or a coffee cup because she remembered putting it down on the table. The solution we came up with was to make three-dimensional versions of the rectangles devised by Robert Efron that we described in Chapter 1—a set of rectangular wooden blocks that varied in width but not in overall area (Figure 2.5). We already guessed, of course, that Dee would have great difficulty distinguishing between these different shapes.

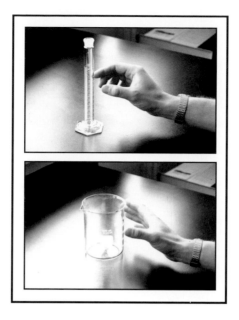

Figure 2.4 Not only do we rotate our hand in the correct orientation as we reach out to grasp an object, but the opening between our thumb and fingers is scaled to the object's size. Thus, we open our hand wider in flight to pick up a beaker than we do to pick up a measuring cylinder.

BOX 2.1 MODELS OF REACHING AND GRASPING

Pioneering work by the late Marc Jeannerod on grasping showed that the movement of the hand towards the goal object (the "transport component") is relatively independent from the formation of the grasp itself (the "grip component"). He demonstrated that changing the size of the goal object led to corresponding changes in grip size but had no effect on the velocity of the moving hand. But when goal objects were placed at different distances from the grasping hand, the velocity of the reach increased for movements of greater amplitude while grip size was largely unaffected. Jeannerod concluded from these findings that the transport and grip components of a grasping movement are generated by independent "visuomotor channels." This so-called "dual channel" hypothesis has become the dominant model of human prehension. Even though later studies have shown that the transport and grip components may be more integrated than Jeannerod originally proposed, there is broad consensus that the two components show a good deal of functional independence.

But Jeannerod's dual channel hypothesis has not gone unchallenged. Jeroen Smeets and Eli Brenner, two researchers based in Amsterdam, have proposed that the movements of each finger of a grasping hand are controlled independently—each digit being simultaneously directed to a different location on the goal object. According to their account, when people

(Continued)

reach out to pick up an object with a "precision" grip, for example, the index finger is directed to one side of the object and the thumb to the other. The apparent scaling of the grip to object size is nothing more than a by-product of the fact that the index finger and thumb are moving towards their respective end points. Moreover, because both digits are attached to the same limb, the so-called transport component is simply the combined movement of the two digits towards the object. Simply put, it is the location in space of the two edges of the object rather than the size of the object that drives grasping—so there is no need to separate grasping into transport and grip components that are each sensitive to different visual cues.

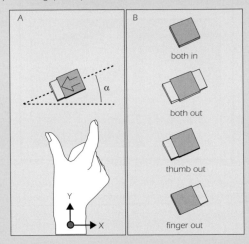

Although Smeets and Brenner's "double-pointing" hypothesis would appear to have the virtue of parsimony, it cannot account for a number of other observations about grasping. For example, Cornelis van de Kamp and Frank Zaal, also based in the Netherlands, have shown that when one side of an object but not the other is suddenly pushed in or out (with a hidden compressed-air device) as people are reaching out to pick it up (see box figure), the trajectories of both digits are adjusted in flight. Smeets and Brenner's model would not predict this. According to their double-pointing hypothesis, only the digit going to the perturbed side of the goal object should change course. But the fact that the trajectories of both digits show an adjustment is entirely consistent with Jeannerod's dual-channel hypothesis. In other words, as the object changes size, so does the grip. Moreover, as we shall see later, the organization of the brain areas involved in the control of reaching and grasping is far more consistent with the dual-channel than it is with the double-pointing hypothesis. Reproduced from *Experimental Brain Research, 182* (1), 2007, 27–34, Prehension is really reaching and grasping, Cornelis van de Kamp, Figure 1, With kind permission from Springer Science and Business Media.

REFERENCES

Jeannerod, M. (1986). Mechanisms of visuomotor coordination: a study in normal and brain-damaged subjects. *Neuropsychologia, 24,* 41–78.

Smeets, J.B.J. and Brenner, E. (1999). A new view on grasping. *Motor Control, 3,* 237–271.

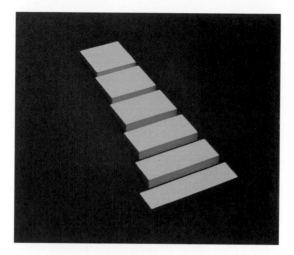

Figure 2.5 "Efron blocks"—these are three-dimensional versions of the Efron rectangles we intro-duced in Chapter 1, Figure 1.9.

In order to monitor the movements of the hand and fingers as the grasp unfolded, we were able to take advantage of new technology that had been developed in Canada. The technique involved attaching tiny infrared lights to the tips of the index finger and thumb. The three-dimensional coordinates of these lights could then be tracked with infrared-sensitive cameras and stored in a computer as the hand moved out to pick up a target object (see Figure 2.6). Special computer soft-ware could then be used to plot how the finger postures changed as the hand moved toward its goal (Figure 2.7). These techniques were already in use in the visuomotor laboratory at the University of Western Ontario where one of us (Mel Goodale) was working.

So in the spring of 1990, Dee and Carlo made their first trip to Canada, spend-ing a week visiting London, Ontario. We gave Dee a day or two to get over her jet lag, and then we brought her into the laboratory where we carried out our first test using the "Efron blocks." Small infrared lights were attached with adhesive tape to Dee's fingers, thumb, and wrist. We placed the shapes in front of her, one by one, and asked her simply to reach out and pick them up and put them down again. When we tracked how she opened her hand as she reached toward the object, we found that she showed exactly the same scaling of her grip "mid-flight" as the normally sighted individuals we tested. In other words, the wider the block, the wider her hand opened (see Figure 2.8). It was clear that like anyone else, she was unconsciously using visual information to program her grasp, and doing so with considerable precision.

25

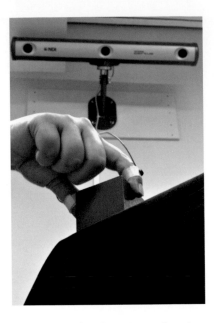

Figure 2.6 This picture shows the small infrared-emitting markers that can be attached to the ends of the finger and thumb. These markers are tracked with infrared-sensitive cameras (shown in the background).

As expected, however, Dee found it difficult to distinguish between these solid rectangles when they were presented as pairs. She could not even show us how wide each block was by using her finger and thumb, which we were able to monitor using the same recording equipment we had used to track her grasping movements. For most people, of course, making such size estimates with the finger and thumb is a simple thing to do. But it was not for Dee, as can be seen in Figure 2.8. Her estimates were wildly inaccurate, and showed no relationship at all to the real width of the blocks. Yet she understood perfectly well what we were asking her to do—when we asked her to imagine a familiar object, like a golf ball or a grapefruit, she had no trouble showing us how big that object was using her finger and thumb.

Of course there are other differences between grasping an object and estimating its size. One difference that has been remarked on recently by Thomas Schenk, a researcher based in Germany, is that only when grasping the blocks did Dee actually get feedback (through touch) about the true size of each block. So perhaps this is how she got to do as well as she did, while her manual estimates were so poor. But of course we had randomly alternated the sequence of blocks we presented to her, so her tactile feedback from grasping one block would have been useless to her when

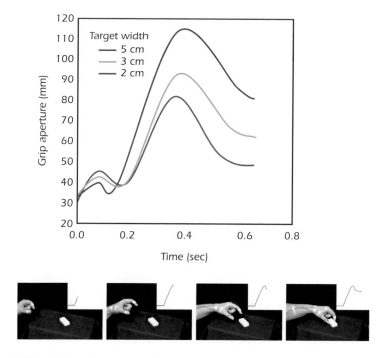

Figure 2.7 Use of infrared movement tracking technology allows us to measure with some precision the change in the grip aperture as the grasping movement unfolds (see sequence of photographs at bottom). As can be seen from the graph at the top, the hand opens to a maximum extent about 70 percent of the way through the reach, and this maximum grip aperture (MGA) is closely related to the width of the goal object: the larger the object, the bigger the MGA.

grasping the next one. So we arrive at a similar conclusion as before: Dee seems to have no trouble in using visual information to program her grasping. Yet, at the same time, she does not have any conscious visual experience of the dimensions of the objects she is picking up so skillfully.

Grasping shape

Dee can deal proficiently with the size and orientation of objects when she has to use those features in making simple behavioral actions. But what about their *shape*? Could she use the outline of an object, the very thing whose absence robs her visual experience of its essential structure, to guide her actions? For example, the rectangular shapes we had used earlier to probe her ability to scale her grasp varied not only in width but also in shape. In this earlier study, the blocks had always been placed

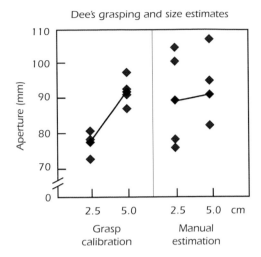

Figure 2.8 The left half of this figure shows the Dee's maximum grip aperture (MGA) during reaching to pick up the narrowest and widest of the Efron blocks. Just like a visually normal person, her MGA is scaled to the width of the blocks. In contrast, as can be seen on the right, Dee is quite unable to indicate (even manually) the width of each block, her estimates varying widely from trial to trial, as if she were guessing. In both halves of the figure, the red diamonds represent separate responses and the black diamonds show her average responses.

in the same orientation and she had been instructed to pick them up front to back. This meant she did not have to use the shape—only the width—to pick up the blocks successfully. But what if they were placed in unpredictable orientations from one occasion to the next and she was given no instructions as to how to pick them up?

When our colleague David Carey carried out a test like this, Dee did just as well as she had done when the blocks were always in the same orientation (see Figure 2.9). This meant her brain must have processed not only the dimensions of the object but also its orientation. In other words, she had to scale her grasp and at the same time rotate her wrist in flight to get her finger and thumb in the right positions. We noticed as well that she nearly always picked up the blocks widthwise rather than lengthwise, even though we gave her no instructions to do this. Obviously, we will pick up a square block equally often either way, because the length is the same as the width. Less obviously, but perhaps not unreasonably, the more elongated the block, the more we go for the width in preference to the length (other things being equal). Dee is no exception to this. This simple fact shows that the undamaged part of Dee's visual brain can not only tailor her grasp to one of the dimensions of the block, but it can work out which dimension is the lesser of the two. This computation then

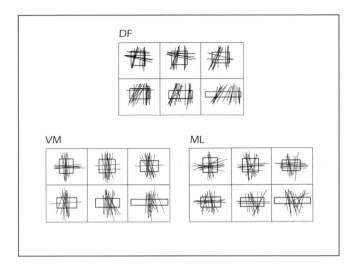

Figure 2.9 These diagrams show how Dee and two healthy control subjects picked up blocks placed in different orientations on a table in front of them. The lines connect the points where the index finger and thumb first made contact with the block. (The results at the different orientations are all shown together on a standard drawing of each block.) Just like the control subjects, when Dee reached out to pick up the block that was nearly square, she was as likely to pick it up lengthwise as widthwise. But with more elongated blocks, she and the control subjects were progressively less likely to do that. None of subjects ever tried to pick up the most elongated block lengthwise. In short, Dee was able to take both the orientation and the shape of the block into account in planning her movement, just like people with normal vision. Reprinted from *Neuropsychologia*, *34*(5), D.P. Carey, M. Harvey, and A.D. Milner, Visuomotor sensitivity for shape and orientation in a patient with visual form agnosia, pp. 329–337, Figure 3. © (1996), with permission from Elsevier.

allows her to choose the most appropriate grasp points, generally at right angles to the principal axis of the shape. In short, her actions can still be guided to some degree by visual shape.

But we were interested to go further and find out whether Dee's visuomotor system could do more than simply compute the dimensions and orientation of regular objects. For many shapes, the visuomotor system must also take into account other geometric properties, such as the curvature of the object at different points around its edges. This is a problem that roboticists have had to address in the development of control systems for so-called "autonomous" robots that can work in unfamiliar environments. In such situations, the robots will often be required to pick up objects that neither they nor their programmer could have anticipated. To do this, the robot, like the human, has to use its optical sensors to compute not only the object's width, orientation, and principal axis, but also the curvature at different places around the object's boundaries. Only by computing the convexities and concavities around the object, would the robot (or the human) be able to select the most stable grasp points—points where the robot's grippers (or the human's finger and thumb) could clasp the object securely.

Discussions with a German colleague, Heinrich Bülthoff, brought to our attention the work of Andrew Blake, an engineer at the University of Oxford, UK. Blake had developed a series of abstract shapes to evaluate the performance of different computer programs he had designed to guide robotic grasping of novel objects. With Bülthoff's help we constructed what we came to refer to as the "Blake shapes," a set of smooth, flat, pebble-like objects, for testing Dee's ability to select stable grasp points on unfamiliar shapes.

When we presented these shapes one by one to Dee, she had no difficulty whatever in picking them up (see Figure 2.10). As she reached to pick up each Blake shape, she made subtle adjustments in the positioning of her finger and thumb in flight so that they engaged the object at stable grasp points on its boundary. Just like people with normal vision, or one of Blake's robots, she would choose stable points the first time she was presented with each object. Yet, needless to say, she was totally

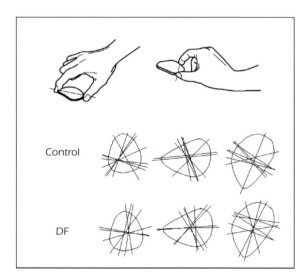

Figure 2.10 The Blake shapes. The drawings at the top show a stable (on the left) and an unstable (on the right) grasp for these irregular shapes. For shapes of this kind, the lines joining the index finger and thumb for a correct grasp would pass through the center of the shape and would be positioned on stable points on the edge of the shape. As the grasp lines shown on the outlines of three typical shapes illustrate, Dee grasped the shapes just as well as the control subject. Reprinted from *Current Biology*, 4(7), Melvyn A. Goodale, John Paul Meenan, Heinrich H. Bülthoff, David A. Nicolle, Kelly J. Murphy, and Carolynn I. Racicot, Separate neural pathways for the visual analysis of object shape in perception and prehension, pp. 604–610, Figure 5, © (1994), with permission from Elsevier.

30

at a loss when it came to saying whether pairs of these smooth objects were alike or different.

Getting around

As we saw at the beginning of this chapter, Dee is able to hike over difficult terrain as skillfully as the next person. When walking through a room, she never bumps into furniture or doorways. In fact, this apparently normal navigation through her immediate environment, coupled with her ability to reach out and shake your hand or take objects that are offered to her, makes many people who meet her for the first time doubt that she has any visual problems at all. She talks to them intelligently about her journey and she even appears to recognize people she knows in the laboratory. As a result, some colleagues who have come to test her have initially been so skeptical as to feel they were wasting their time—they could test such an apparently normal person any time!

Of course, as all psychologists should know, appearances can be deceiving. For example, Dee's recognition of people that she has met on previous occasions need not be due to any visual ability, but rather to her ability to remember what someone's voice sounds like. (Though it is true that she can use certain visual cues, like color. We had a colleague in St Andrews with a penchant for dyeing his hair bright colors—often more than one. Dee never had any difficulty recognizing him.) A skeptic (as psychologists are by nature) could argue likewise that in the anecdote with which we started this chapter, Dee's ability to negotiate the trail at Monrosa might owe much to her previous experience with this popular picnic spot.

So we needed a way to test her ability to walk around an unfamiliar environment, in which we could specify beforehand the precise nature of the obstacles placed in her path. Fortunately, at the University of Waterloo, only an hour away from the University of Western Ontario, a colleague of ours, Aftab Patla, was studying just this kind of locomotor skill in people with normal vision. Patla had constructed a special laboratory in which he could place obstacles of particular heights at specified points along a route that his volunteers were asked to follow. With the help of the same kind of opto-electronic equipment that we were using at Western, he was able to measure the adjustments that people automatically make to their gait as they step over such obstacles.

On one of Dee's several visits to Canada, we drove her to Waterloo where she was quite happy to try Patla's test. She walked through his test environment absolutely confidently and without tripping over any of the obstacles, which varied in height from less than an inch up to fifteen inches (see Figure 2.11). In fact, her behavior was indistinguishable from that of other volunteers. Just like them, she effortlessly raised

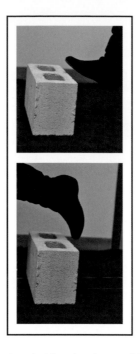

Figure 2.11 A foot going over an obstacle. Note that the toe of the leading foot just clears the top of the obstacle; the same is true for the toe of the trailing foot as well. In other words, we leave just enough clearance to make sure that our foot doesn't touch the obstacle—rather than leaving a large safety margin.

her foot just enough to clear each of the obstacles. It will come as no surprise to the reader, however, that when asked to estimate the height of the obstacles in a separate test, Dee was much less accurate than the normal volunteers.

How does she do it?

All the laboratory testing confirmed our informal observations: in one sense, Dee sees perfectly well. She uses visual information about the size, the orientation, and to some degree the shape, of objects to execute skilled movements. Yet in another sense, Dee sees nothing at all—and can certainly tell us nothing—about the attributes of the goal objects.

So what was the essential difference between the situations in which she succeeded and those where she failed? As pointed out earlier, it is not simply the case that she is unable to put her visual experience into words. Nor is it the case that whenever she makes some kind of skilled limb movement in response to a visible object she gets it right. Take, for example, the posting test. Her ability to insert the card into the slot cannot simply be put down to the fact that she was making a manual action. She had to make a hand movement in the matching test as well—yet she failed completely. The critical difference therefore is not that a movement was made in one case but not in the other. It is the purpose of the movement that matters. When we asked people to use their hand to show us what they saw in the matching test, they were reporting on their conscious perception of the slot in front of them. Turning the hand in this case was an act of communication. The fact that the communication happened to be manual was arbitrary—the same information could have been conveyed by a variety of different means. They could have drawn a line on piece of paper, for example; or picked the correct orientation from a number of alternatives in a multiple choice test; or of course they could simply have told us in words. Dee could do none of these things—not because she couldn't communicate—but because she had nothing visual to communicate. She had no conscious experience, no conscious visual experience at least, of the orientation of the slot to share with us.

The action that Dee had to make in the original posting test had a very different purpose. To get the card into the slot, she had no choice but to turn her hand in a particular direction. This rotation was an obligatory part of the action rather than being an arbitrary act of communication. Dee had to make the same kind of rotation of her wrist when she reached out to pick up a rectangular block or a pencil placed at a particular orientation. Such movements are part of an ancient repertoire that we share with our present-day primate cousins, the monkeys and apes, and presumably also with our own primate ancestors. For example, when we are standing in a crowded subway train and it suddenly jerks to a stop, we may find ourselves quickly reaching out to grasp a handrail to steady ourselves. We do this without thinking, yet our brain has to do some complex processing so that our hand can turn rapidly and accurately so as to grasp the rail. This echoes the kinds of unthinking hand movements our arboreal ancestors would have had to make when grasping branches and when foraging for food.

The most amazing thing about Dee is that she is able to use visual properties of objects such as their orientation, size, and shape, to guide a range of skilled actions—despite having no conscious awareness of those same visual properties. This contrast between what she can and cannot do with visual information has important implications about how the brain deals with incoming visual signals. It indicates that some parts of the brain (which we have good reason to believe are badly damaged in Dee) play a critical role in giving us visual awareness of the world while other parts (relatively undamaged in her) are more concerned with the immediate visual control of skilled actions.

Perhaps this should not be too surprising. On the one hand we need vision for the online control of everyday actions—particularly for those actions where speed is at a premium and we have no time to think. But on the other hand we also need vision to make sense of the world around us when we do have time to think! In fact, for most people, including most vision scientists, this perceptual experience of the world is the most important aspect of vision. What perception does for us is to translate the ever-changing array of "pixels" on our retina into a stable world of objects that exists independent of ourselves. This allows us to construct an internal model of the external world that enables us to attach meaning and significance to objects and events, to understand their causal relations, and to remember them from day to day. Perception also allows us to plan our future actions, and to communicate with others about what we see around us.

Summary

Our studies with Dee highlight the two distinct jobs that vision does for us: the control of action on the one hand, and the construction of our perceptual representations on the other. As we will see in the next two chapters, these two different functions of vision have shaped the way the visual brain has evolved. Rather than evolving some kind of general-purpose visual system that does everything, the brain has opted for two quite separate visual systems: one that guides our actions and another, quite separate, system that handles our perception.

Thinking about vision this way certainly helps us to understand Dee's predicament. The anoxic episode (see Chapter 1, Box 1.1) profoundly affected her vision for perception but left her vision for action largely unscathed. What was lucky for us as scientists, and also of course for her, was that the damage was so specific that her vision-for-action system has continued to operate remarkably successfully in isolation. What the damage did was to uncover in Dee a system that we all use, but one that is normally overshadowed and outshone by our concurrent visual experience of the world. Her tragic accident has allowed us to bring this visuomotor system out of the shadows, and to explore its operating characteristics and scope.

Further Reading

These two early publications describe our first discoveries of Dee's spared visual abilities and deficits:

Goodale, M.A., Milner, A.D., Jakobson, L.S., and Carey, D.P. (1991). A neurological dissociation between perceiving objects and grasping them. *Nature, 349,* 154–156.

Milner, A.D., Perrett, D.I., Johnston, R.S., Benson, P.J., Jordan, T.R., Heeley, D.W., Bettucci, D., Mortara, F., Mutani, R., Terazzi, E., and Davidson, D.L.W. (1991). Perception and action in "visual form agnosia". *Brain*, *114*, 405–428.

Further developments were published in these two subsequent articles:

Carey, D.P., Harvey, M., and Milner, A.D. (1996). Visuomotor sensitivity for shape and orientation in a patient with visual form agnosia. *Neuropsychologia*, *34*, 329–338.

Goodale, M.A., Meenan, J.P., Bülthoff, H.H., Nicolle, D.A., Murphy, K.J., and Racicot, C.I. (1994). Separate neural pathways for the visual analysis of object shape in perception and prehension. *Current Biology*, *4*, 604–610.

III

When vision for action fails

The startling visual dissociations we have described in Dee Fletcher point to the existence of two relatively independent visual systems within the brain— one for conscious perception, which is severely damaged in Dee, and another for the unconscious control of action, which is largely preserved. But skeptics could argue that all we have documented in Dee is a case of someone with poor vision. Maybe you do not need as much visual information to guide your actions as you do to perceive and recognize people and objects. Dee's vision might be good enough for picking something up, but not good enough for telling what it is. In other words, maybe there is only one visual system, not two, and in Dee's case it is simply functioning below some threshold level. On the face of it, this is a tenable argument. But if it were true, then there shouldn't be any cases of brain-injured individuals who show the *opposite* pattern of deficits and spared visual abilities to that seen in Dee. It should always be conscious perception that suffers first. Yet as we shall see in this chapter, such patients do exist. Moreover, the part of the visual brain that is damaged in these individuals is quite different from that damaged in Dee.

Bálint's syndrome

Even at the beginning of the 20th century, neurologists were describing cases of patients whose visual problems could be more accurately characterized as *visuomotor* in nature. In other words, they were describing cases where a patient had a specific problem in translating vision into action. Later work has gone on to show that at least some of these patients show remarkably intact visual perception—despite having profound difficulties performing even the simplest visually guided movements. In short, the clinical picture they present is the mirror image of Dee Fletcher's.

The Hungarian neurologist Rudolph Bálint was the first to document a patient with this kind of problem, in 1909. The patient was a middle-aged man who suffered a massive stroke to both sides of the brain in a region called the parietal lobe (see Chapter 1, Figure 1.10). Although the man complained of problems with his eyesight, he certainly was not agnosic in the way that Lissauer's and Freud's patients were. He could recognize objects and people, and could read a newspaper. He did tend to ignore objects on his left side and had some difficulty moving his eyes from one object to another. But his big problem was not a failure to recognize objects, but rather an inability to reach out and pick them up. Instead of reaching directly toward an object, he would grope in its general direction much like a blind man, often missing it by a few inches. Unlike a blind man, however, he could see the object perfectly well—he just couldn't guide his hand toward it. Bálint coined the term "optic ataxia" (*optische Ataxie*) to refer to this problem in visually guided reaching.

Bálint's first thought was that this difficulty in reaching toward objects might be due to a general failure in his patient to locate where the objects were in his field of vision. But it turned out that the patient showed the problem only when he used his right hand. When he used his left hand to reach for the same object, his reaches were pretty accurate. This means that there could not have been a generalized problem in *seeing* where something was. The patient's visual processing of spatial location per se was not impaired. After further testing, Bálint discovered that the man's reaching difficulty was not a purely motor problem either—some kind of generalized difficulty in moving his right arm correctly. He deduced this from asking the patient to point to different parts of his own body using his right hand with his eyes closed: there was no problem.

So the optic ataxia that Bálint's patient suffered from was a truly "visuomotor" disorder, in the sense that the patient could not use visual information about the location of the target specifically to guide his (right) arm toward that target. That is, although the disorder affected behavior directed at visual targets, it could not be explained away as a general problem in either visuospatial processing or motor control. Unfortunately, this important conclusion has been largely overlooked by subsequent generations of neurologists, particularly in the English-speaking world. This may have been partly because Bálint's report remained untranslated for many years. Instead, most British and North American neurologists have followed the influential English physician and scientist Gordon Holmes, and attributed these kinds of reaching difficulties to a general disorder in visuospatial perception. This disorder was assumed to affect all aspects of behavior that are dependent on the spatial locations of objects in the visual field.

What has gone wrong in optic ataxia?

It was not until the 1980s that research on patients with optic ataxia was kick-started again, mostly by Marc Jeannerod and his group in Lyon, France. In one landmark study, his colleagues Marie-Thérèse Perenin and Alain Vighetto made detailed video recordings of a sizeable group of patients with optic ataxia performing a number of different visuomotor tests. They were thus the first investigators to measure and analyze quantitatively the errors that these patients make in reaching toward target objects placed in different spatial locations. Like Bálint, they observed that although their patients couldn't accurately point to the targets, they were able to give pretty accurate verbal reports of where those same objects were located. Also like Bálint, Perenin and Vighetto demonstrated that the patients had no difficulty in directing hand movements toward different parts of their own body. Subsequent work in their laboratory went on to show that the reaching and pointing errors made by many patients with optic ataxia are most severe when they are not looking directly at the target. But even when pointing at a target in the center of the visual field, the patients still make bigger errors than normal people do, albeit now on the order of millimeters rather than centimeters. In short, Perenin and Vighetto's research confirms Bálint's original conclusion: optic ataxia is a deficit in visually guided reaching, not a general deficit in spatial vision.

Like most researchers at that time, Perenin and Vighetto studied reaching behavior by stripping the task down to its essential core, with a stationary target object presented on an otherwise empty table. But of course in everyday life the situation is rarely that simple, and Perenin and Vighetto's pioneering studies have led subsequent researchers to explore more complex scenarios. For instance, when we reach for an object, our brain generally has to take account not only of where that particular target object is—it also has to take account of other objects in the vicinity to make sure we don't collide with them en route. For example when we reach out to pick up our morning cup of coffee at the breakfast table, our hand generally finds its way to the cup without hitting the glass of orange juice in the process—the hand automatically takes a path that reduces the chances of any such collision.

Avoiding potential collisions during reaching turns out to be a real problem for patients with optic ataxia. To get a handle on this aspect of reaching, our colleague Robert McIntosh designed a simple test in which he asked people to make a series of reaches from a fixed starting point toward a clearly marked strip 25 cm away across the table (see Figure 3.1, left). The only complication was that their reaches had to

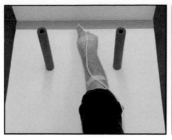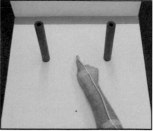

Figure 3.1 The apparatus we used for testing obstacle avoidance during reaching. The picture on the left shows a person reaching between two cylinders to touch a gray strip at the back of the board. On the right, the person is being asked to point to the midpoint between the two cylinders. In the first case the person is not asked explicitly to "bisect" the space between the two cylinders, but simply to make a natural movement toward the goal (the gray strip). The second task is quite different: here the person is asked to give an explicit judgment about the space between the two cylinders by making a pointing movement to the midpoint between them.

pass between two vertical rubber cylinders, each of which could appear in either of two slightly different locations. There was little danger of an actual collision with either of these cylinders, as they were always separated by at least 16 cm. Yet virtually everyone we have ever tested, including a range of brain-damaged patients, has consistently varied the line of their reach, slightly to the left or the right, according to the positions of these potential obstacles. In fact the only exception has been patients with optic ataxia, every one of whom has failed to make these automatic adjustments to their reach trajectories.

We first discovered this when we tested two patients in Lyon in collaboration with our French colleagues. One of the patients, Anne Thiérry, has a large area of damage to the parietal lobe on both sides of the brain, very much like Bálint's original case. The second patient, Irène Guitton, is 20 years younger than Anne, and she too has damage to both parietal lobes, though much more restricted in extent. Both Anne and Irène suffer from a similarly severe optic ataxia, but Irène's lesser damage frees her from the other aspects of Bálint's syndrome, such as a failure to make eye movements to scan the visual environment. Yet despite their differences, neither patient showed any sign of adjusting their reaching movements in McIntosh's task to take into account the positions of the potential obstacles (see top half of Figure 3.2). Irrespective of where the cylinders were placed, they each moved their finger toward the gray strip along the same route every time.

The absence of the normal side-to-side adjustments in Anne's and Irène's reaches cannot be explained away as a failure to see the varying positions of the two cylinders. When they were asked to make judgments of the midpoint between the

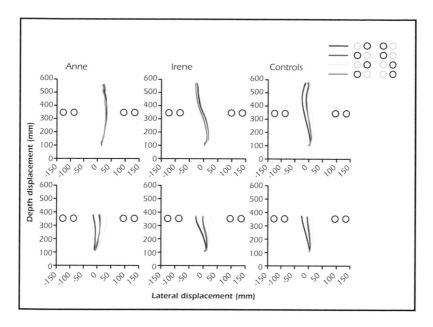

Figure 3.2 The top diagram shows the average reaches made by Anne and Irène across the four different configurations of the two cylinders (the average routes for these four different configurations are represented by different colors). Both patients follow the same route whatever the locations of the two cylinders used in the experiment (shown as circles). In contrast, healthy volunteers ("controls") automatically shift their routes rightwards or leftwards in a systematic fashion (top right). As shown in the bottom diagram, neither Anne nor Irène has any trouble indicating the midpoint between the two cylinders as their positions changed from one reach to the next. In fact their behavior is indistinguishable from that of the controls. Adapted with permission from Macmillan Publishers Ltd: *Nature Neuroscience*, 7(7), Igor Schindler, Nichola J. Rice, Robert D. McIntosh, Yves Rossetti, Alain Vighetto, *et al.*, Automatic avoidance of obstacles is a dorsal stream function: evidence from optic ataxia, 779–784, Figure 3. © 2004.

cylinders (by pointing to it; see Figure 3.1, right) they followed the changes in position of the cylinders from side to side just like our control subjects did (see bottom half of Figure 3.2). So their unvarying reaches are not caused by a failure to *see* the potential obstacles, but instead reflect a failure to incorporate what they see into their movements—just like their primary problem, directing reaches to a target whose location they can see perfectly well.

A few years later, we embarked on a series of tests with another optic ataxia patient, Morris Harvey. Unlike Anne or Irène, Morris has damage in only one of his parietal lobes, his left one. This has resulted in an optic ataxia that is highly selective—it is present only when he uses his right hand, and only when reaching toward targets in his right side of space. Nichola Rice-Cohen, then a graduate student working in our labs, was interested to see how Morris would deal with obstacles. She found that when Morris reached with his left hand, he behaved quite normally, shifting his route according to the positions of the two cylinders. But things changed dramatically when he used his right hand. Remarkably, he now took absolutely no account of the obstacle on the right, even though he continued to respond to the one on the left. So it seems that Morris's brain damage has selectively interfered with the visual control of right-hand reaching, but only when the target for the reach, *or any potential obstacle*, is located in his right visual field.

The apparently simple job of reaching out to a target can present other problems as well for patients with optic ataxia. One problem has been particularly well documented in the case of Irène Guitton. Our French colleagues Laure Pisella and Yves Rossetti had Irène make a series of reaches to touch a small LED target. From time to time, however, the target would unpredictably shift leftwards or rightwards at the very instant Irène's hand started to move toward it. Healthy volunteers doing this task had no problem in making the necessary in-flight corrections to their reach, and in fact they adjusted their reaches seamlessly as if their movements were on "automatic pilot," particularly when under time pressure to move quickly. Yet Irène found these changes in target location frustratingly impossible to deal with. It was as if she no longer had that automatic pilot. To put it another way, Irène's reaches seemed to be entirely predetermined at the outset of the movement, and remained impervious to unexpected changes in the position of the target, even though she could see them clearly enough and knew they might occur. On occasions when the target moved, she found herself reaching first to its original location, and only then shifting her finger to the new location.

Of course in everyday life, cups of coffee do not capriciously shift their location just as we reach out for them. But our brains evolved not just to enable us pick up stationary objects like cups, but to let us grab moving targets as well—such as small prey animals or fruit on a branch that is blowing in the wind. Not only that—*we* move too, not just our potential targets. So faced with these challenges, the brain seems to have evolved a system where the hand first heads in the general direction of a target, but is then able to correct itself en route, using visual feedback about the relative positions of the hand and the target. This online self-correction system is apparently lost in Irène Guitton.

All of these studies converge in helping us to characterize what has gone wrong in optic ataxia. In one study after another, starting with Perenin and Vighetto's work, we see the same pattern emerging. First we see that the patients can describe the location of the objects to which they can't accurately reach. Then we find that they are fully aware of the location of potential obstacles but somehow cannot avoid them when reaching to a target. And finally we discover that these patients can perceive a sudden shift in the position of a target but cannot adjust their moving hand online to accommodate the shift. In short, in all these cases we see a clear dissociation between "spatial perception" and "spatial action." That is, optic ataxia patients can *perceive* the full set of visual information they need to use—they just can't *act* upon that perceived information. So Bálint was right. Optic ataxia is a *visuomotor* deficit—in a more comprehensive sense than he ever envisaged—and not, as Gordon Holmes maintained, part of a larger overarching deficit in spatial perception.

Other difficulties associated with optic ataxia

In one of their pioneering tests during the 1980s, Marie-Thérèse Perenin and Alain Vighetto examined the ability of their patients to reach out and pass their hand through an open slot cut in a disk, which could be positioned at different orientations at random (see Figure 3.3). Remarkably, not only did the patients tend to make the expected spatial errors, in which their hand missed the slot altogether, but they also made orientation errors, in which the hand would approach the slot at the wrong angle. Yet most of these same patients could easily tell one orientation of the slot from another when asked to do so. So again we see a familiar story unfolding. The failure of the patients to rotate their hand as they reached out to pass it through a slot was not due to a difficulty in perceiving the orientation of the slot—the problem was visuomotor in nature, not perceptual. (Of course when their hand made

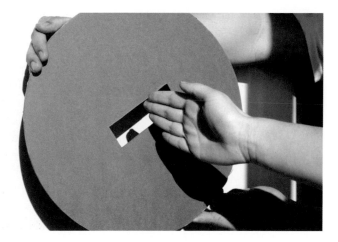

Figure 3.3 Marie-Thérèse Perenin and Alain Vighetto discovered that patients with "optic ataxia" not only have problems reaching to point to something accurately, but also tend to direct their hand at the wrong angle when trying to pass it through a slot. The same patients, however, often have no problem describing the orientation of the slot in words.

contact with the disk they could correct themselves using touch, and then pass their hand through the slot. In other words the deficit was restricted to the modality of sight, and did not extend to touch.)

As described in Chapter 2, it was by borrowing Perenin and Vighetto's slot task that we were first able to provide a convincing demonstration of Dee Fletcher's pre-served visuomotor abilities in the context of her profound visual form agnosia. In other words, Dee's pattern of performance on the slot task nicely complements the earlier work with optic ataxia patients. The next question is, does this neat contrast between the two kinds of patients also extend to the other tests we found Dee to be good at, such as grasping objects of different sizes?

Again the relevant evidence was gathered in France, in this case by Marc Jeannerod, who, as we noted in Chapter 2, pioneered the application of quanti-tative methods to the analysis of visually guided grasping in healthy volunteers. Importantly, Jeannerod went on to show that the well-regulated patterns of move-ment that typify a normal person's reaching and grasping behavior were severely disrupted in patients with optic ataxia. Instead of first opening the hand during the early part of the reach, and then gradually closing it as it moved toward the target object, the optic ataxia patient would keep the hand widely opened throughout the movement, much as a person would do if reaching blindfolded toward the object (see Figure 3.4). Jeannerod and his colleagues were the first to carry out systematic tests with Anne Thiérry, the optic ataxia patient we described earlier in this chapter. They used similar matching and grasping tasks to those we had used earlier with Dee (see Chapter 2). Anne was found to show poor scaling of her grip when reaching for objects of different sizes, while remaining well able to demonstrate the sizes of the objects by use of her forefinger and thumb. Again, the pattern of deficits and spared abilities in Anne and the pattern in Dee complement each other perfectly.

The work we have summarized so far shows that optic ataxia patients not only have problems directing their actions to visual targets in space, but they also have trouble with other visuomotor tasks in which object size and orientation are the critical factors. At the same time, when asked to *distinguish between* objects on the basis of their size, orientation, or relative location, many of these patients do quite well. As we saw, this pattern of behavior is the converse of what we found with Dee. And it doesn't end there. We tested an optic ataxia patient called Ruth Vickers with the "Blake" shapes described in Chapter 2. We were interested to see whether she would show the opposite pattern of results to that shown by Dee.

Ruth was a middle-aged woman from a small town in rural Canada, who had recently suffered two strokes, one on each side of the brain, the second stroke occurring within a week of the first. Brain imaging showed that the damage was almost symmetrically located in the parietal lobe, again rather like Bálint's patient

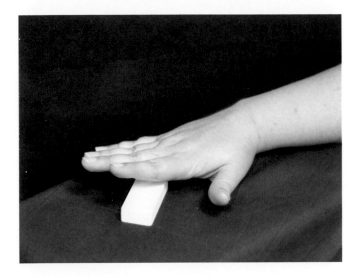

Figure 3.4 A typical example of a poor grip in a patient with optic ataxia. Her posture resembles someone groping in the dark for an object they know is there, although in this case the patient can see the object perfectly well. Of course as soon as the hand makes contact with the goal object, the person uses touch to close the hand and form a normal grasp.

(see Figure 3.5). Her clinical picture initially looked very much like that described by Bálint. Although Ruth's symptoms had cleared to some degree by the time we saw her, it was obvious that she still had severe optic ataxia. She could not reach with any degree of accuracy to objects that she could see but was not looking at directly. She could, however, reach reasonably accurately to objects directly in her line of sight.

Nevertheless, the reaches Ruth made to pick up an object she was looking at, although spatially accurate, were far from normal. Like Anne Thiérry, she would open her hand wide as she reached out, no matter how big or small the objects were, showing none of the grip scaling seen in healthy people (see Figure 3.6). Yet despite this, when asked to show us how big she thought the object was using her finger and thumb, she performed quite creditably, again just like Anne. And she could describe most of the objects and pictures we showed her without any difficulty. In fact, although her strokes had left her unable to control a pencil or pen very well, she could draw quite recognizable copies of pictures she was shown (see Figure 3.7). In other words, Ruth's visual experience of the world seemed pretty intact, and she could readily convey to us what she saw—in complete contrast to Dee Fletcher.

Because Ruth could distinguish between many different shapes and patterns, we did not expect her to have much difficulty with the smooth pebble-like shapes we had tested Dee with earlier. We were right—when she was presented with a pair

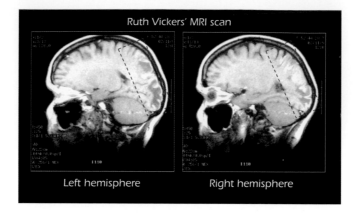

Figure 3.5 MRI scan of Ruth Vickers' brain showing a "slice" from front to back through each half of the brain. The white areas at the back show the degenerated tissue on both sides of the brain resulting from Ruth's two strokes. The damaged areas can be clearly seen within the red rectangles.

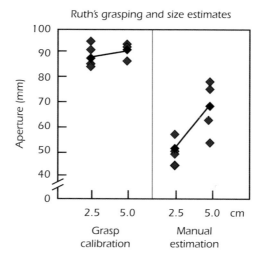

Figure 3.6 The right half of this figure shows Ruth's manual estimates of the widths of the narrowest and widest of the Efron blocks. The red diamonds represent separate responses and the black diamonds the mean of all the responses. Although she shows more variability than healthy people, her estimates show that she can clearly see the difference between the two blocks. Indeed, her verbal descriptions are quite normal. Despite her good *perception* of what blocks look like, she fails to scale her grip to the width of the blocks, and instead opens her hand widely on all occasions using a splayed-hand posture (see Figure 3.4). Note the contrast between Ruth's pattern of performance with Dee's as shown in Figure 2.8.

Model   Copy

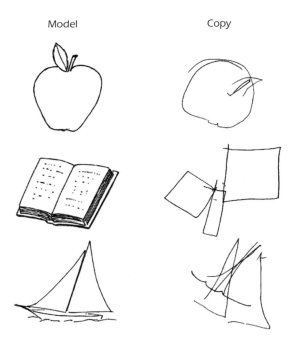

Figure 3.7 Unlike Dee, Ruth Vickers had no difficulty recognizing and naming the drawings shown on the left. Even when she was asked to copy them (right), she was able to capture many of the features of the drawings. Nonetheless it is obvious that she had difficulties coordinating her movements as she did her drawings.

of "Blake shapes" she could generally tell us whether or not the two shapes were the same. Although she sometimes made mistakes, particularly when two identical shapes were presented in different orientations, her performance was much better than Dee's. When it came to picking up the shapes, however, the opposite was the case. Ruth had real problems. Instead of gripping the Blake shapes at stable "grasp points," she positioned her finger and thumb almost at random (see Figure 3.8). This inevitably meant that after her fingers contacted the pebble she had to correct her grip by means of touch—if she did not, the pebble would often slip from her grasp. In other words, although some part of Ruth's brain could code the shape of these objects to inform her visual experience, her hand was unable to use such shape information to guide its actions.

The upshot of all this research is that patients who develop optic ataxia after parietal lobe damage are liable to have other visuomotor problems as well. That is, their deficits typically go beyond a failure to reach accurately towards a point in space. Indeed many patients show visuomotor difficulties that are not about an object's location in space at all. For example, they don't rotate their wrist or open their grasp appropriately when picking up objects. And Ruth Vickers couldn't direct her grasp to the appropriate points on the edges of the object that she was trying to pick up. In other words, misreaching in space is just one part of a spectrum of deficits in visual guidance of action that damage to the parietal lobes can cause. So not only do patients with optic ataxia show a deficit in visually guided reaching, as Bálint argued, but they frequently have a range of other visuomotor disorders as well (Box 3.1).

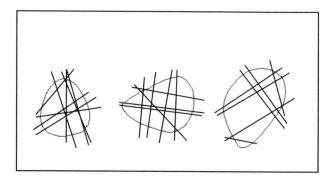

Figure 3.8 Examples of Ruth's attempts to pick up "Blake" shapes. Unlike Dee (see Chapter 2), she often grasped the shapes at inappropriate points, so that the shape would slip out of her fingers. Reprinted from *Current Biology*, 4(7), Melvyn A. Goodale, John Paul Meenan, Heinrich H. Bülthoff, David A. Nicolle, Kelly J. Murphy, and Carolynn I. Racicot, Separate neural pathways for the visual analysis of object shape in perception and prehension, pp. 604–610, Figure 5. © (1994), with permission from Elsevier.

BOX 3.1 SPATIAL NEGLECT AND APRAXIA

The parietal lobes (numbered "2" in Figure 1.10 in Chapter 1) encompass a large area of the surface of the brain, extending from the side, right over the top, and down into the inner (medial) surface facing the other hemisphere. So it should come as no surprise that damage to different parts of the parietal lobe can result in quite different problems for the patient. The areas lower down at the sides (the "inferior parietal lobule," IPL) are frequently damaged as a consequence of major stroke, when the middle cerebral artery on one side is disrupted or blocked, depriving a large area of brain tissue of its oxygen lifeline. When this happens, usually the patients do not have the kinds of visuomotor symptoms seen in optic ataxia, but they do have problems that may at first sight seem related. These problems are different depending on which side the damage is on.

The typical result when a stroke affects the IPL on the *right* side of the brain, is that the patient suddenly starts to pay little or no attention to things on her left side—almost as if that side of the world no longer exists for her. This condition is known as "spatial neglect," and is illustrated

(Continued)

in the figure in this box. In this patient, studied by Valerie Brown in our lab, the brain damage was caused by a hemorrhage in the parieto-temporal part of the right hemisphere, as shown in the computed tomography scan at the top. The patient tended to neglect the leftward parts of lines he was asked to bisect, marking them to the right of center (bottom left); he tended to miss leftward-lying random lines after being asked to mark them all (bottom middle); and he tended to miss left-sided details of a drawing he was asked to copy (bottom right).

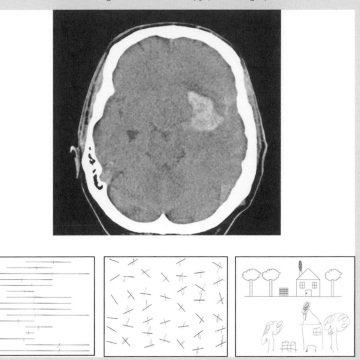

Spatial neglect can present quite serious difficulties for rehabilitating the patient's other symptoms, such as hemiparesis, in which the limbs on the left side become weak or paralyzed. In patients with full Bálint's syndrome, this area is damaged *as well as* the superior part that causes optic ataxia. It is partially damaged in Anne Thiérry but not in Irène Guitton. The important point is that damage to the IPL alone can cause spatial neglect but will not cause optic ataxia, while lesions restricted to the superior parietal region can cause optic ataxia but will not cause spatial neglect. The two disorders are quite distinct in both their cause and their nature.

Curiously, damage to the IPL on the *left* typically does not cause neglect—instead it can cause a condition known as apraxia. The disorder in apraxia is neither visual nor spatial in nature, but affects the planning and execution of actions. A typical problem that such a person may have is a difficulty in miming how to use a particular implement, such as a toothbrush. As before of course, a large area of left parietal damage may cause both optic ataxia *and* apraxia, but again the two typically occur separately, according to whether the damage affects the superior or inferior parts of the parietal lobe.

So two patients, Anne and Ruth, show a pattern of spared abilities and deficits that is the exact converse of the pattern we observed in Dee with respect to the shape and size of objects. What about the other way around? Would Dee perform well on some of the tests of obstacle avoidance, for example, that present problems for optic ataxia patients? Given that Dee retains good visuomotor control in a range of situations, our expectation was that she would do equally well on Rob McIntosh's obstacle avoidance task. We already knew that she had little trouble avoiding obstacles when walking in an unfamiliar street or room, and as we saw in Chapter 2 she translated this into a normal performance when negotiating the experimental "obstacle course" in Aftab Patla's lab in Canada. Informally, we also knew that she could avoid obstacles when reaching out to pick up an object from a cluttered desk or table—provided, of course, that she has already identified the goal object, either because it has a distinctive color or because it has been flagged in some other way. At dinner, for example, we had observed her reaching to pick up her glass of wine without bumping into other things on the table—even when it meant that her reaching hand had to take a circuitous route to do this. But of course we couldn't be sure whether she did this by memorizing the position of the wine glass and nearby objects—or whether she was adjusting her movements automatically in the same way as she avoids a chair or coffee table when walking around in an unfamiliar room. In fact, we had never actually tested Dee's ability to avoid obstacles when reaching out for objects in the laboratory. When we went ahead and tested her on Rob McIntosh's reaching task, we found that she did quite well, avoiding the obstacles just as well as some of the normal volunteers we tested. In contrast, she performed poorly when asked to indicate the midpoint between the two obstacles. Dee's active avoidance of the obstacles despite her imperfect perception of their location is the exact opposite of the performance of our optic ataxia patients, Anne and Irène, who show no sign of reacting to obstacles whose location they clearly perceive.

Summary

We have seen in this chapter that, in many different respects, optic ataxia patients present a quite opposite pattern of visual disabilities (and spared visual abilities) to the pattern we saw in Dee Fletcher. This has important theoretical implications for our interpretation of what is going on in the brains of these different patients. Going back to the concern with which we began this chapter, it cannot simply be the case that brain damage degrades the quality of Dee's visual experience in an undifferentiated way, so that some tasks can still be done while other "more difficult" ones cannot. If this were true, then optic ataxia patients like Ruth and Anne should show the same pattern of deficits and spared abilities as Dee. But of course they show the opposite. There is no way that a unitary general-purpose visual system can explain this.

Conversely, the fact that Dee Fletcher shows intact visuomotor control in the face of a profound perceptual loss also undercuts a commonsense account of what causes optic ataxia. Some scientists have argued that optic ataxia is simply a "disconnection" between visual perception and action, in which the perceptual information just cannot get through to the motor system. According to this intuitively reasonable view, there is only one kind of visual processing, which not only provides our conscious perception, but also the visual guidance for all our actions. But if this were the case, then how could Dee, whose visual perception of object form has been lost, carry out actions based on object form? If she does not have the perception, she should not be able to perform the visually guided actions that putatively depend on that perception. In short, Dee's spared abilities disprove this disconnection account of optic ataxia.

The existence of opposite patterns of lost and spared abilities in two kinds of brain damage is known in the trade as a "double dissociation." What a double dissociation like this one shows is that when brain damage impairs one task (a recognition test, for example) but not another (such as a test of visuomotor skill), that difference cannot simply be put down to the second task being easier than the first. The other half of the double dissociation (in this case a visuomotor impairment coexisting with intact visual perception) rules that out. What double dissociations can also suggest—but cannot strictly prove—is that different, quasi-independent brain systems (or brain "modules" as they are sometimes called) are handling each of the two abilities that are dissociated. In the present instance, there is certainly prima facie evidence for this. Dee's brain damage, as the reader may recall from Chapter 1, is chiefly concentrated in the occipito-temporal region, whereas, in contrast, the optic ataxia patients we have been discussing in this chapter invariably have had damage in the parietal lobes (see Figure 1.10). In other words, the evidence so far points to the idea that the occipito-temporal region may be associated with visual perception of the world, whereas the parietal lobe may be more important for the visual guidance of action. But developing this argument further requires independent and converging evidence from other kinds of brain research. In Chapter 4 we will discuss some of the relevant evidence, beginning with a discussion of the evolution of vision in the vertebrate brain and the emergence of modularity.

Further Reading

The first description of optic ataxia is given in this classic paper by Rudolph Bálint, translated into English by Monika Harvey:

Harvey, M. (1995). Translation of "Psychic paralysis of gaze, optic ataxia, and spatial disorder of attention" by Rudolph Bálint. *Cognitive Neuropsychology*, *12*, 261–282.

The critical role of the parietal lobe in visuomotor control was confirmed experimentally in a group of optic ataxia patients in the following paper, published nearly 80 years after Bálint's original case report:

Perenin, M.-T. and Vighetto, A. (1988). Optic ataxia: a specific disruption in visuomotor mechanisms. I. Different aspects of the deficit in reaching for objects. *Brain*, *111*, 643–674.

A comprehensive review of work on the neural substrates of the visually guided action, including descriptions of the reaching and grasping deficits in optic ataxia, can be found in:

Jeannerod, M. (1997). *The Cognitive Neuroscience of Action*. Oxford: Blackwell.

For details of the work on obstacle avoidance during reaching in patients with brain damage in the dorsal or ventral streams, see:

Rice, N.J., McIntosh, R.D., Schindler, I., Mon-Williams, M., Démonet, J.-F., and Milner, A.D. (2006). Intact automatic avoidance of obstacles in patients with visual form agnosia. *Experimental Brain Research*, *174*, 176–188.

Schindler, I., Rice, N.J., McIntosh, R.D., Rossetti, Y., Vighetto, A., and Milner, A.D. (2004). Automatic avoidance of obstacles is a dorsal stream function: evidence from optic ataxia. *Nature Neuroscience*, *7*, 779–784.

IV

The origins of vision: from modules to models

For most of us, sight is our pre-eminent sense. We don't just *respond* to the patterns of light on our retina: we *experience* them. We experience them as integral components of a visual world that has depth, substance, and most important of all, a continuing existence separate from ourselves. It is through visual experience that we gain most of our knowledge about external reality, and the possession of that knowledge, in turn, powerfully affects the way we see other things. In fact visual knowledge determines much of the basic content of our consciousness. Visual knowledge allows us to plan future actions, to picture the consequences of those actions, and to re-live (sometimes with pleasure, sometimes with regret) what we have seen and done in the past. Vision affects the way we feel, as well as the way we think. Visual experiences can evoke powerful emotions, both positive and negative—as can the visual memories of what we have experienced before. Given the importance of vision in our mental life, it is not surprising that our language is full of visual metaphors. We can "see the point," if we are not "blind to the facts"; and occasionally show "foresight" (though perhaps more often "hindsight") by "seeing the consequences" of our actions in our "mind's eye."

It is tempting to think that the delivery of such vivid experiences and the knowledge they impart is the entire raison d'être for vision. But the visual brain did not begin—in evolutionary terms—as a system designed to deliver conscious visual experience. That aspect of vision, while clearly extremely important, is a relative newcomer on the evolutionary landscape. So how did vision begin?

To answer this question, we have to turn to evolutionary biology and ask: "What is vision good for?" The answer from a biological point of view is quite straightforward. Vision evolved only because it somehow improved an animal's fitness—in other words, improved its ability to survive and reproduce. Natural selection, the differential survival of individuals in a population, ultimately depends on what animals *do* with the vision they have, not on what they *experience*. It must have been the case therefore that vision began, in the mists of evolutionary time, as a way of guiding an organism's behavior. It was the practical effectiveness of our ancestors' behavior that shaped the ways our eyes and brains evolved. There was never any selection pressure for internal "picture shows"—only for what vision could do in the service of external action. This is not to say that visual thinking, visual knowledge, and even visual experience did not arise through natural selection. But the only way this could have happened is through the benefits these mental processes provide for behavior. Before returning to the intricacies of human vision, let us consider for a moment what kind of a role vision plays in the lives of simpler organisms, which presumably do not have any mental life at all.

The origins of vision

A single-cell organism like the *Euglena*, which lives in ponds and uses light as a source of energy, changes its pattern of swimming according to the different levels of illumination it encounters in its watery world. Such behavior keeps *Euglena* in regions of the pond where an important resource, sunlight, is available. But although this behavior is controlled by light, no one would seriously argue that the *Euglena* "sees" the light or that it has some sort of internal model of the outside world. The simplest and most obvious way to understand this behavior is that it works as a simple reflex, translating light levels into changes in the rate and direction of swimming. Of course, a mechanism of this sort, although activated by light, is far less complicated than the visual systems of multicellular organisms. But even in complex organisms like vertebrates, many aspects of vision can be understood entirely as systems for controlling movement, without reference to perceptual experience or to any general-purpose representation of the outside world.

Vertebrates have a broad range of different visually guided behaviors. What is surprising is that these different patterns of activity are governed by quite independent visual control systems. The neurobiologist, David Ingle, for example, showed during the 1970s that when frogs catch prey they use a quite separate visuomotor "module" from the one that guides them around visual obstacles blocking their path. These modules run on parallel tracks from the eye right through the brain to the motor output systems that execute the behavior. Ingle demonstrated the existence

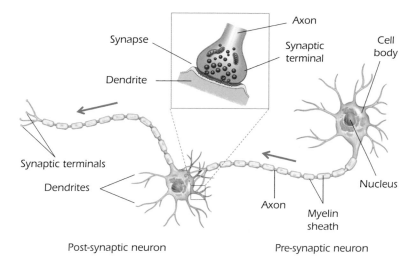

Figure 4.1 A schematic diagram of two neurons. The right-hand one is sending signals to the one on the left. Information coded as electrochemical changes in the cell membrane flows within the cell from the dendrites (from the Greek for "branches") and the cell body to the axon. The inset shows the synapse—the gap between the two communicating neurons. Information flows from the pre-synaptic axon at the top to the post-synaptic dendrite below, using chemical transmission. The myelin forms a discontinuous white fatty sheath that insulates the axon and speeds up transmission. Bundles of axons form the so-called "white matter" of the brain, whereas aggregations of cell bodies form the "gray matter."

of these modules by taking advantage of the fact that nerves (bundles of axons; see Figure 4.1) in the frog's brain, unlike those in the mammalian brain, can regenerate new connections when damaged. In his experiments, he was able to "rewire" the visuomotor module for prey catching by first removing a structure called the optic tectum on one side. The optic nerves that brought information from the eye to the optic tectum on the damaged side of the brain were severed by this surgery. A few weeks later, however, the cut nerves re-grew, but finding their normal destination missing, crossed back over and connected with the remaining optic tectum on the other side of the brain. As a result, when these "rewired" frogs were later tested with artificial prey objects, they turned and snapped their tongue to catch the prey—but *in the opposite direction* (see Figure 4.2). This "mirror-image" behavior reflected the fact that the prey-catching system in these frogs was now wired up the wrong way around.

But this did not mean that their entire visual world was reversed. When Ingle tested the same frogs' ability to jump around a barrier blocking their route, their movements remained quite normal, even when the edge of the barrier was located

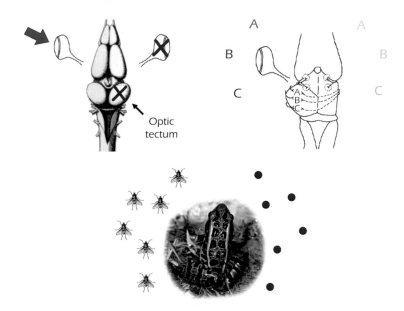

Optic tectum

Figure 4.2 This figure illustrates a critical experiment by David Ingle. As the upper left drawing shows, Ingle removed the optic tectum on one side of the frog's brain and the eye that normally projected to the remaining optic tectum. Initially, the frog appeared to be blind and did not "snap" at prey items. Some weeks later, however, when artificial prey (shown as flies) were presented at different locations to the eye opposite the missing optic tectum, the frog snapped at mirror-image points on the other side (shown as red circles). This is because the eye had become hooked up in a systematic way to the optic tectum on the wrong side of the brain (see drawing upper right). The optic tectum interprets the signals from this eye as if they were coming from the missing eye (its usual source of visual input). In other words, prey items presented to the eye at points A, B, and C were treated as if they were coming from the mirror-image locations on the blind side (indicated by the faint A, B, and C). From David Ingle, Two visual systems in the frog, *Science*, *181*(4104), 1053–1055, Figure 1. © 1973 The American Association for the Advancement of Science. Reprinted with permission from AAAS.

in the same part of space where they made prey-catching errors (see Figure 4.3). It was as though the frogs saw the world correctly when skirting around a barrier, but saw the world mirror-imaged when snapping at prey. In fact, Ingle discovered that the optic nerves were still hooked up normally to a separate "obstacle avoidance module" in a part of the brain quite separate from the optic tectum. This part of the brain, which sits just in front of optic tectum, is called the pretectum. Ingle was subsequently able to selectively rewire the pretectum itself in another group of frogs. These animals jumped right into an obstacle placed in front of them instead of avoiding it, yet still continued to show normal prey catching.

So what did these rewired frogs "see"? There is no sensible answer to this. The question only makes sense if you believe that the brain has a single visual

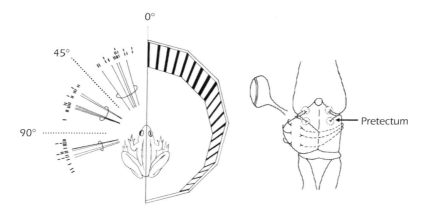

Figure 4.3 This diagram shows the directions in which the "rewired" frog jumped in response to a gentle touch from behind in the presence of a barrier. The barrier was sometimes extended beyond the midline to positions 45° or 90° into the visual field of the rewired eye. A successful escape required the frog to turn and jump just enough to clear the edge of the barrier. The rewired frogs always cleared the barrier successfully, just like normal frogs. This is because only the eye's projections to the optic tectum were rewired: the other projections, including those to the pretectum, which supports barrier avoidance behavior, remained correctly hooked up. From David Ingle, Two visual systems in the frog, *Science*, *181*(4104), 1053–1055, Figure 1. © 1973 The American Association for the Advancement of Science. Reprinted with permission from AAAS.

representation of the outside world that governs all of an animal's behavior. Ingle's experiments reveal that this cannot possibly be true. Once you accept that there are separate visuomotor modules in the brain of the frog, the puzzle disappears. We now know that there are at least five separate visuomotor modules in the brains of frogs and toads, each looking after a different kind of visually guided behavior and each having distinct input and output pathways. Obviously the outputs of these different modules have to be coordinated, but in no sense are they all guided by a single visual representation of the world residing somewhere in the frog's brain.

The same kind of visuomotor "modularity" exists in mammals as well. Evidence for this can be seen even in the anatomy of the visual system. As Box 4.1 makes clear, the nerve cells (neurons) in the retina send information (via the optic nerve) directly to a number of different sites in the brain. Each of these brain structures in turn gives rise to a distinctive set of outgoing connections. The existence of these separate input–output lines in the mammalian brain suggests that they may each be responsible for controlling a different kind of behavior—in much the same way as they are in the frog. The mammalian brain is more complex than that of the frog, but the same principles of modularity still seem to apply. In rats and gerbils, for example, orientation movements of the head and eyes toward morsels of food are governed by brain circuits that are quite separate from those dealing with obstacles that need to be avoided while the animal is running around. In fact, each of these brain circuits in the mammal shares a common ancestor with the circuits we have already mentioned in frogs and toads. For example, the circuit controlling orientation movements of the head and eyes in rats and gerbils involves the optic tectum (or "superior colliculus" as it is called in mammals), the same structure in the frog that controls turning and snapping the tongue at flies.

BOX 4.1 ROUTES FROM THE EYE TO THE MAMMALIAN BRAIN

Neurons in the retina send information along the optic nerve to a number of distinct target areas in the brain. The two largest pathways within the optic nerve are the ones projecting to the superior colliculus (SC) and the dorsal part of the lateral geniculate nucleus in the thalamus (LGNd). The pathway to the SC is a much more ancient system (in the evolutionary sense) and is the most prominent pathway in other vertebrates such as amphibians, reptiles, and birds. The SC (or optic tectum, as it is called in non-mammalian animals) is a layered structure forming the roof (Latin: *tectum*) of the midbrain. It is interconnected with a large number of other brain structures, including motor nuclei in the brainstem and spinal cord. It also passes information to a number of different sites in the cerebral cortex. The SC appears to play an essential role in the control of the rapid eye and head movements that animals make toward important or interesting objects in their visual world.

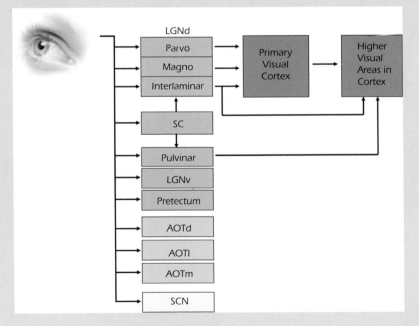

(Continued)

The pathway to the LGNd is the most prominent visual pathway in humans and other higher mammals. Neurons in the primate LGNd project in turn to the cerebral cortex, with almost all of their axons ending up in the primary visual area, or striate cortex (often nowadays termed area V1) in the occipital lobe. This set of projections and its cortical elaborations probably constitute the best-studied neural system in the whole of neuroscience. Scientists' fascination with the so-called "geniculo–striate" pathway is related to the fact that our subjective experience of the world depends on the integrity of this projection system (see the section entitled "Blindsight" in Chapter 6).

Although the projections to the SC and LGNd are the most prominent visual pathways in the human brain, there are a number of other retinal pathways that are not nearly so well studied as the first two. One of the earliest pathways to leave the optic nerve consists of a small bundle of fibers that project to the so-called suprachiasmatic nucleus (SCN). The visual inputs to the SCN are important for synchronizing our biorhythms with the day–night cycle.

There are also projections to the ventral portion of the lateral geniculate nucleus (LGNv), the pulvinar nucleus and various pretectal nuclei, and a set of three nuclei in the brainstem known collectively as the nuclei of the accessory optic tract (AOT). The different functions of these various projections are not yet well understood—although they appear to play a critical role in the mediation of a number of "automatic" reactions to visual stimuli. The AOT have been implicated in the visual control of posture and certain aspects of locomotion, and have been shown to be sensitive to the "optic flow" on the retina that is created as we move through the world. The AOT also plays an important role in controlling the alternating fast and slow eye movements that we make when looking at a large visual stimulus, such as a train, passing before our eyes. Retinal projections to one area in the pretectum are thought to be part of the circuitry controlling the pupillary light reflex—the constriction of the pupil as we move into a brightly lit environment such as the beach or the ski slopes. There is also some evidence from studies in amphibians and lower mammals that certain pretectal nuclei play a role in visually guided obstacle avoidance during locomotion, as we saw earlier in this chapter. However almost nothing is known about the functions of other pretectal nuclei, the ventral part of the lateral geniculate nucleus, or the pulvinar.

The fact that each part of the animal's behavioral repertoire has its own separate visual control system refutes the common assumption that all behavior is controlled by a single, general-purpose representation of the visual world. Instead, it seems, vision evolved, not as a single system that allowed organisms to "see" the world, but as an expanding collection of relatively independent visuomotor modules.

Vision for perception

Of course, in complex animals such as humans and other primates like monkeys, vision has evolved well beyond this set of discrete visuomotor modules. Much of our own behavior is certainly not rigidly bound to our current sensory input. Even frogs can learn to some degree from their previous visual encounters with the world—but humans and other higher primates can use their previous visual experience and knowledge of the visual world in much more flexible ways to guide what they do in the future. We can internally rehearse different courses of action, for example, often using visual imagery in doing so, before deciding what to do.

In other words, vision can serve action not just in the here and now, but also "offline"—at other times and in other places. To do this, the visual brain creates a rich and detailed representation of the visual scene that the animal is looking at. We don't know what animals experience, but in humans at least, these perceptual representations are normally conscious. We experience them, and thereby we can communicate them to others. The visual mechanisms that generate these representations are quite different from the simple visuomotor modules of frogs described earlier, and have almost certainly arisen more recently in evolutionary time. Rather than being linked directly to specific motor outputs, these new mechanisms create a perceptual representation that can be used for many different purposes. Moreover, as we mentioned in Chapter 1, our perception of the world is not slavishly driven by the pattern of light on the eye but is also shaped by our memories, emotions, and expectations. Visuomotor mechanisms may be driven largely "bottom-up" but perception has an important "top-down" component as well. The memories that affect our perception in this top-down way are themselves built up from previous perceptions. As a result of all this two-way traffic, perception and memory literally blend into one another. After all, we have visual experiences in our dreams, and these must be generated entirely by top-down processes derived from memory.

These general-purpose representations confer a big advantage in that they allow us to choose a goal, plan ahead, and decide upon a course of action. But on the other hand they do not have any *direct* contact with the motor system. The "online" visual control of our actions still remains the responsibility of dedicated visuomotor modules that are similar in principle to those found in frogs and toads.

It is important to bear in mind that when people talk about what they "see," they are talking only about the products of their perceptual system. Until recently even scientists studying human vision have seen no need to go further than perceptual reports when gathering their data. In fact, an important tradition in visual research called "psychophysics" depends entirely on what people report about what they can and cannot see. It has always been assumed that this is all there is to vision. Admittedly, psychophysics, which was founded by the 19th-century German physicist-turned-philosopher, Gustav Fechner, has told us a great deal about the capacities and limits of the perceptual system. But it has told us nothing about how vision controls the skilled movements that we make. As our research with Dee shows, the reason that traditional psychophysics has failed in this regard is because the operations of the visuomotor machinery governing our actions are simply not available for conscious report. We may have a conscious visual experience of a coffee cup in front of us, but this experience will tell us little about the particular visual information that enables us to pick up the cup.

Traditional psychophysics, then, can tell us nothing about the ways that visual information controls our movements. For this, we need a new kind of psychophysics, a "visuomotor psychophysics," that looks at the effects of variations in the properties of a visual stimulus, not on what people say they see, but rather on what they actually do. A start on this enterprise has been made by our Israeli colleague Tzvi Ganel (see Box 4.2).

BOX 4.2 DIFFERENT PSYCHOPHYSICS FOR PERCEPTION AND ACTION

The 19th-century German physician and scientist, Ernst Heinrich Weber, is usually credited with the observation that our sensitivity to changes in any physical property or dimension of an object or sensory stimulus decreases as magnitude of that property or dimension increases. For example, if a bag of sugar weighs only 50 grams, then we will notice a change in weight if a only few grams of sugar are added or taken away. But if the bag weighs 500 grams, much more sugar must be added or taken away before we notice the difference. Typically, if the weight of something is doubled, then the smallest difference in weight that can be perceived is also doubled. Similar, but not identical, functions have been demonstrated for the loudness of sounds and the brightness of visual stimuli. In short, the magnitude of the "just-noticeable difference" (JND) increases with the magnitude or intensity of the stimulus. Gustav Fechner later formalized this basic psychophysical principle mathematically and called it Weber's law.

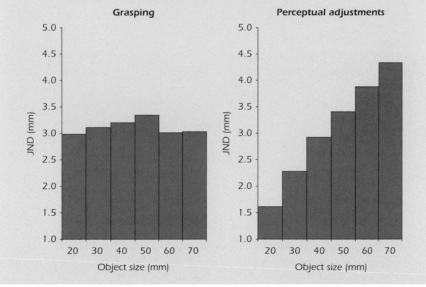

(Continued)

Almost all studies of Weber's law have involved asking observers to *tell* the experimenter about what they see. They do this by giving a report either verbally or manually (by hitting a computer key, for example). But as we have already discussed, vision is also used to guide and shape our actions, and here a fundamentally different psychophysical approach is required— one that measures how our hand movements, for example, are related to the visual features of an object we are trying to pick up. It turns out that this new "visuomotor psychophysics" looks very different from traditional psychophysics. Tzvi Ganel, an Israeli scientist based at Ben-Gurion University of the Negev, has examined what happens to the calibration of grasping when the size of the goal object is manipulated. He and his colleagues found something quite remarkable. Unlike perceptual estimates of object size, grip scaling does not appear to obey Weber's law. When people estimated the size of an object by adjusting a comparison line on a computer screen, the JND increased with physical size just as one would expect from Weber's law. But when people reached out to pick up the object, the JND, as measured by differences in grip aperture, was unaffected by variations in the size of the object (see box figure). In other words, visually guided actions appear to violate Weber's law, reflecting a fundamental difference in the way that object size is computed for action and for perception. We will revisit this issue in Chapters 7 and 8.

REFERENCE

Ganel, T., Chajut, E., and Algom, D. (2008). Visual coding for action violates fundamental psychophysical principles. *Current Biology, 18,* R599–R601.

Vision for action

Alongside the evolution of perceptual systems in the brains of higher mammals such as humans, the visuomotor systems in turn have become progressively more complex. The main reason for this is that the movements we make have become more complex. In our primate ancestors, one of the great landmarks in evolution was the emergence of the prehensile hand—a device that is capable of grasping objects and manipulating them with great dexterity. But just as the development of any sophisticated piece of machinery, such as an industrial robot, needs an equally sophisticated computer to control it, the evolution of the primate hand would have been useless without the co-evolution of an equally intricate control system. The control of eye movements too has become more sophisticated and has become closely linked with the control of our hand movements. All of these changes, in other words, were accompanied by the evolution of new brain circuitry. Many of these new control systems in the brain have strong links to and from the basic modules in those older parts of the brain that were already present in simpler vertebrates like the ancestors of frogs and toads. As Ganel's experiments show us (see Box 4.2), the computations that these visuomotor circuits carry out seem to be quite different from those supporting perception.

A good example of the way that these more recently evolved circuits operate can be seen in the control of the rapid ("saccadic") eye movements that humans and other primates use to explore their visual environment. We saw already that head and eye movements in rodents are controlled by the same basic structures (the optic tectum, or superior colliculus) that control prey-catching in frogs. These structures retain a central role in the machinery that programs saccadic eye movements in primates as well. But now these ancient visuomotor circuits have become subject to regulation and refinement by newer brain structures in the cerebral cortex (the outer rind of gray matter that forms the evolutionary pinnacle of the brain), where more intricate computations can be brought into play.

At first sight this may seem a puzzle—why didn't nature devise totally new systems from the ground up? In his book *Evolving Brains*, the American neurobiologist John Allman tells the story of how, on a visit to a power generation plant during the 1970s, he was struck by the side-by-side coexistence of several control systems for the generators dating from different periods in the life of the plant. There were pneumatic controls and a system of controls based on vacuum tube technology, along with several generations of computer-based control systems. All of these systems were being used to control the processes of electrical generation at the plant. When he asked the reason for this strange mix, he was told that the demand for power had always been too great for the plant ever to be shut down. As Allman points out:

> The brain has evolved in the same manner as the control systems in this power plant. The brain, like the power plant, can never be shut down and fundamentally reconfigured, even between generations. All the old control systems must remain in place, and new ones with additional capacities are added and integrated in such a way as to enhance survival.

It seems, however, that while these expanded visuomotor systems in higher mammals govern much more complex behaviors, they remain essentially automatic and are no more accessible to consciousness than those in the frog (or in *Euglena* for that matter). They might carry out more sophisticated and subtle computations on the visual information they receive, but they can do this perfectly well without a visual "representation" of the world. In fact, these visuomotor networks no more need conscious representations of the world than does an industrial robot. The primary role of perception is not in the *execution* of actions, but rather in helping the person or animal to arrive at a decision to act in a particular way.

As we shall now see in the last section of this chapter, there has been a massive expansion in primates of the areas devoted to visual processing in the most prominent part of the mammalian brain—the cerebral cortex. We can understand this development by seeing it as reflecting the two closely related developments that we have outlined earlier. One development is the emergence of *perceptual systems* for identifying objects in the visual world and attaching meaning and significance to them. And the other is the emergence of more complex *visuomotor control systems* that permit the execution of skilled actions directed at those objects.

The sites of sight: two visual streams in the primate cortex

In 1982, a seminal article appeared in the literature that has been cited more frequently than any other paper in the field of visual neuroscience, before or since. It was called "Two cortical visual systems" and was written by two eminent American neuroscientists, Leslie Ungerleider and Mortimer Mishkin. They summarized converging experimental evidence mostly derived from monkeys, whose visual brains and visual abilities are closely similar to ours. Signals from the eyes first arrive at the cerebral cortex in a small area at the back called the primary visual area (V1). Ungerleider and Mishkin argued convincingly that the signals were then routed forwards along two quite separate pathways within the cortex (see Figure 4.4). One of these routes, which they called the dorsal visual pathway, ended up in part of the brain at the top of the cerebral hemispheres, the posterior parietal region. The other (the so-called ventral visual pathway) ended up at the bottom and sides of the hemispheres, in the inferior temporal region. These two pathways are now often called the dorsal and ventral *streams* of visual processing.

Many more visual areas have been discovered in the thirty years since then, and as a result we now know that there is a far more complicated pattern of interconnections than anyone thought possible back in 1982 (see Figure 4.5). Nevertheless, the basic wiring plan first identified by Ungerleider and Mishkin still stands: a dorsal stream going to the posterior parietal cortex and a ventral stream going to the inferior temporal cortex. It was ten years after their initial description of the two pathways that we suddenly realized what the division of labor between these two information highways in the monkey's brain might be. In a light-bulb moment, we could see that the division maps rather neatly onto the distinction between "vision for action" and "vision for perception" in humans that we have been we have just described.

The basic experimental evidence for this functional distinction between the two streams comes from two complementary kinds of research in monkeys. First, there

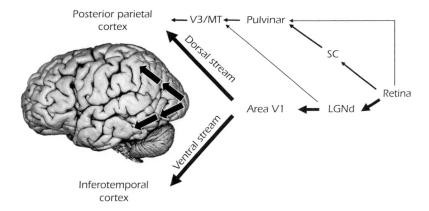

Figure 4.4 A schematic diagram of the two streams of visual processing in primate cerebral cortex. The ventral stream receives nearly all of its visual input from the primary visual cortex (V1), which in turn receives its input from the lateral geniculate nucleus (LGNd) of the thalamus. The dorsal stream also receives input from V1, but in addition gets substantial inputs from the superior colliculus (SC) via the pulvinar (Pulv), another nucleus in the thalamus. This pathway and others shown on the diagram remain intact in patients who have damage to V1, with important consequences, as we shall see in Chapter 6. The arrows on the inset photograph of the human brain show the approximate route of the two streams within the cerebral hemispheres.

is evidence from lesion experiments, in which the dorsal and ventral streams in monkeys have been separately damaged to see what effects this damage might have on different kinds of visual behavior. Second, there is evidence from single-cell recording, in which the kinds of visual information that are encoded in individual nerve cells (neurons) can be monitored.

Doing without one stream

Studying how brain damage affects behavior in animals has had a long history. Even in mid-Victorian times, experimentally minded neurologists had begun to make selective lesions of brain tissue in animals, in the hope of gaining some understanding of the many brain-damaged people entering their clinics. The Scottish neurologist David Ferrier was a pioneer in this field. During the 1860s, he removed what we now call the dorsal stream in a monkey, and discovered that the animal would misreach and fumble for food items set out in front of it. In a similar vein, recent work by Mitchell Glickstein in England has shown that small lesions in the dorsal stream can make a monkey unable to pry food morsels out of narrow slots set at different orientations. The monkey is far from blind, but it cannot use vision to insert its finger and thumb at the right angle to get the food. It eventually does it by touch, but

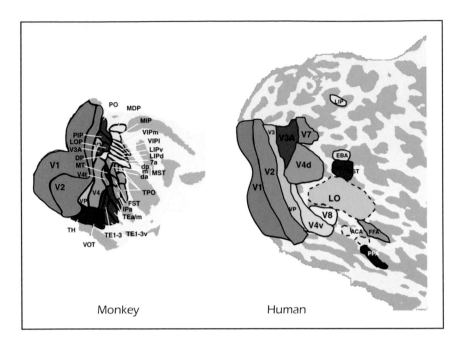

Figure 4.5 A comparison of the layout of visual areas in macaque monkey and human brain, presented as flattened representations of the cortical surface. Areas believed to be homologous in the two species share the same color. Not all of the areas identified in monkey have yet been located in the human brain, but the catching-up process is proceeding fast. The two "flat maps" are of course not shown to the same scale. Reprinted from Tootell, R.B.H., Tsao, D., and Vanduffel, W., Neuroimaging weighs in: humans meet macaques in "primate" visual cortex. *Journal of Neuroscience*, 23, 3981–3989, Figure 1. © 2003, Society for Neuroscience, with permission.

its initial efforts, under visual guidance, fail. Yet the same monkey has no difficulty in telling apart different visual patterns, including lines of different orientation. These observations, and a host of others, have demonstrated that dorsal-stream damage in the monkey results in very similar patterns of disabilities and spared abilities to those we saw in Ruth Vickers and Anne Thiérry. In other words, monkeys with dorsal-stream lesions show major problems in vision for action but evidently not in vision for perception.

In direct contrast, Heinrich Klüver and Paul Bucy, working at the University of Chicago in the 1930s, found that monkeys with lesions of the temporal lobes, including most of what we now know as the ventral stream, did not have any visuomotor problems at all, but did have difficulties in recognizing familiar objects, and in learning to distinguish between new ones. Klüver and Bucy referred to these problems as symptoms of "visual agnosia," and indeed they do look very like the problems that

Dee Fletcher has. Moreover, like Dee, these monkeys with ventral-stream lesions had no problem using their vision to pick up small objects. The influential neuroscientist, Karl Pribram, once noted that monkeys with ventral-stream lesions that had been trained for months to no avail to distinguish between simple visual patterns, would sit in their cages snatching flies out of the air with great dexterity. Mitchell Glickstein recently confirmed that such monkeys do indeed retain excellent visuomotor skills. He found that monkeys with ventral-stream damage had no problem at all using their finger and thumb to retrieve food items embedded in narrow slots—quite unlike his monkeys with dorsal-stream lesions.

Eavesdropping on neurons in the brain

Physiologists had devised methods by the 1950s for recording the electrical activity of individual nerve cells ("neurons") in the living brain (see Figure 4.6). The 1980 Nobel laureates David Hubel and Torsten Wiesel used these techniques to study the visual system while working at Harvard in the late 1950s. Much to their surprise, they found that neurons in primary visual cortex (area V1) would "fire" (i.e. give a small electrical response) every time a visual edge or line was shown to the eye, so long as it was shown at the right orientation and in the right location within the field of view. The small area of the retina where a visual stimulus can activate a given neuron is called the neuron's "receptive field." Hubel and Wiesel discovered, in other words, that these neurons are "encoding" the orientation and position of particular

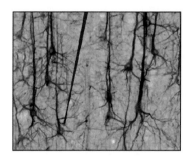
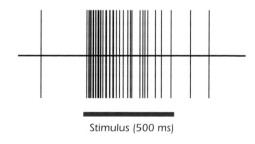

Stimulus (500 ms)

Figure 4.6 The photograph shows the tip of a microelectrode superimposed on a stained section of brain tissue, to show the relative size of the electrode in relation to typical neurons. (In reality the neurons would be much more densely packed than shown here, since only a minority of cells show up using this particular kind of histological stain.) Alongside the photograph is a diagram representing a train of electrical events (action potentials) recorded by such a microelectrode when the adjacent neuron is activated by a suitable visual stimulus. Each vertical line represents a single action potential. Action potentials are discrete events of constant magnitude, like gun shots, forming a digital rather than an analog code for transmitting information along the axon.

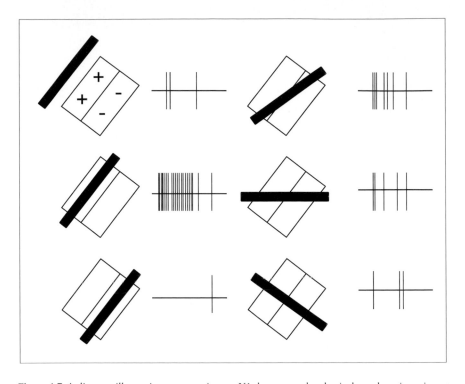

Figure 4.7 A diagram illustrating a neuron in area V1 that responds selectively to the orientation at which an edge or bar is shown to a monkey. The rectangle marks the location in space where the bar has to be presented for the neuron to respond (the neuron's receptive field). The plus signs indicate a region of the receptive field where presenting a small stimulus will result in a burst of firing in the neuron. The negative signs indicate a region where presenting a small stimulus will result in a decrease in firing rate. This means that the orientation of the bar is critical in determining the firing rate of the neuron. Other neurons will have their receptive fields organized differently and thus will "prefer" a different orientation of the bar.

edges that make up a visual scene out there in the world. Different neurons prefer (or are "tuned" to) different orientations of edges (see Figure 4.7). Other neurons are tuned for the colors of objects, and still others code the direction in which an object is moving. The distribution of these neurons within primary visual cortex is not haphazard. Neurons tuned to a particular orientation, for example, are clustered together in "columns," which run through the depth of the cortex. This columnar organization is superimposed on a basic retinotopic layout on the cortical surface of V1 (see Box 4.3), with more area devoted to the central part of the retina than to the rest of the retina. When Hubel and Wiesel explored visual areas beyond primary visual cortex, they found neurons that coded for more complicated visual features.

BOX 4.3 MAPPING THE BODY ONTO THE BRAIN

One interesting feature of brain organization is that the sensory surfaces of the body, including the retina, are mapped in a topographic manner onto the surface of the cortex. Thus, neighboring points on the skin's surface are mapped onto adjacent parts of the cerebral cortex region that processes the sense of touch. The areas of this so-called "somatosensory" cortex that receive input from the hands, for example, are immediately adjacent to those areas receiving input from the arms. Indeed, the surface of the whole body is laid out in a systematic fashion along primary somatosensory cortex from the top of the head to the tips of the toes. Another characteristic of this "somatotopic" map is that those regions of the body that are the most sensitive to touch, such as the fingers, lips, and sex organs, have a much larger amount of cerebral cortex devoted to them than do less sensitive regions such as the trunk. This "cortical magnification" reflects the fact that more sensitive regions of the skin contain more sensory receptors and so require more brain tissue (i.e. neurons) to process the incoming sensory signals. The topographic organization of the somatosensory cortex is often depicted as a sensory "homunculus" (Latin for "little human"), a distorted figure in which the parts of the body that have relatively more sensory neurons than other parts are depicted as larger (see first box figure). A similar topographic organization can be seen in motor cortex, in which more brain tissue is devoted to the fingers, hands, and tongue, for example, than to the trunk and thighs—in this case, reflecting the differences in the dexterity of the motor control exhibited by these different parts of the body.

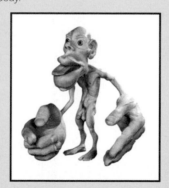

The inputs from the eyes that eventually reach primary visual cortex in the cerebral cortex are also organized in a topographic manner. The half of the retina in each eye that represents the left visual field sends inputs to primary visual cortex in the right hemisphere while the other half (which represents the right visual field) sends inputs to the left hemisphere (see Figure 6.9). In fact, the whole of the visual field is laid out across primary visual cortex in both hemispheres in a so-called "retinotopic" fashion so adjacent neurons process information from adjacent, but overlapping, parts of visual space. As the box figure shows, the central part of the visual field (colored in red) is represented in visual cortex located towards the back of the occipital lobe in both human and monkey, whereas the more peripheral parts of the visual field (colored in blue

(Continued)

and purple) are represented further forward. The central visual field, where our vision is best, occupies the lion's share of the cortical territory—another example of cortical magnification. The first descriptions of maps of the visual field in the human brain were made by Tatsui Inouye, a Japanese ophthalmologist, who observed a relationship between visual field defects (blind areas in the visual field) and the site of brain damage in young soldiers injured in the Russo-Japanese War (1904–1905). Similar observations were made quite independently by Gordon Holmes (see Chapter 3), who examined young men injured in World War I. Later work in both animals and humans has demonstrated that retinotopic maps can be found in many visual areas of the brain. The mapping shown in the second figure in this box, however, was done using sophisticated modern brain imaging in which activity in the intact brain was measured as the monkeys or humans looked at a screen on which moving patterns were systematically presented in different parts of the visual field.

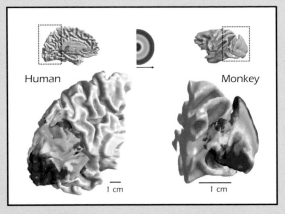

The topographic mapping found in sensory areas of the brain make it easier for neurons receiving input from adjacent regions of the sensory surface to integrate that information. For example, because there is a correspondence between locations on the retina and locations of neurons in primary visual cortex, information about an object in the world that is projected onto the retina will activate neurons in primary visual cortex that are spatially contiguous. As a consequence the exchange of information between these neurons is far more efficient. Similar arguments can be made for the somatosensory system—and indeed for motor control, where the activation of neighboring muscle groups has to be coordinated.

Not surprisingly, sensory systems like hearing, where the computation of the spatial location of sound sources depends on differences in the timing and amplitude of sound arriving at the two ears, show no topographical organization in the cerebral cortex. Interestingly, however, auditory cortex does show a "tonotopic" mapping in which different frequencies of sound are organized in a systematic fashion across the cortical surface.

The 1960s and early 1970s heralded great advances in single-cell recording as investigators pushed well beyond the early visual areas, out into the dorsal and ventral streams. It soon became apparent that neurons in the two streams coded the visual world very differently.

The first person to probe the inferior temporal cortex, deep in the ventral stream, was Charles Gross at Princeton University. He found that neurons here were not satisfied with simple lines and edges, but needed to "see" much more complex visual patterns before they would fire. In fact some neurons were so specific that they remained silent until a hand or a face was presented on the screen in front of the monkey (see Figure 4.8). Keiji Tanaka, a neuroscientist working in Tokyo, found clusters of neurons in inferior temporal cortex analogous to the columns previously found in area V1—only this time the neurons do not share a simple preference like 45°-oriented edges, they share a preference for a particular complex pattern of features. These ventral-stream neurons respond to their preferred visual features over a relatively wide area of the retina. Importantly, however, these large receptive fields almost always include the central and most high-resolution part of the retina (the fovea). In other words, these sophisticated neurons in the ventral stream are focused primarily on that small part of the world where the monkey's eyes are directed at a given moment, and rather less on the rest of the visual field. Even more than area V1,

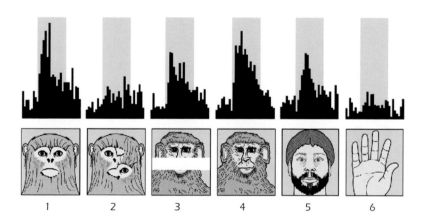

Figure 4.8 An example of a "face cell" recorded within the ventral stream of a monkey's brain. This particular cell responded well to pictures of human or monkey faces seen in full front view, but less well when the picture was jumbled or when other objects such as a hand were shown to the monkey. The responses of the neuron are shown at the top as the total number of action potentials recorded over many test trials, at a series of time points. The gray area on each graph shows the time over which the picture of the face or other object was shown to the monkey. Adapted from *Journal of Cognitive Neuroscience*, 3 (1), Face-selective cells in the temporal cortex of monkeys, Robert Desimone, 1-8 (figure 2) (c) 1991, The MIT Press, with permission.

then, the ventral stream specializes in central vision at the expense of more peripheral parts of the retina. Of course monkeys, like us, can move their eyes around, thereby sweeping the fovea rapidly across the whole scene. By integrating these successive foveal snapshots, the monkey's brain can construct a full representation of the scene in front of the monkey.

Although the neurons in the ventral stream are quite fussy about the kind of object they respond to, a good number of them are quite unfussy about the particular viewpoint from which the object is seen or even where it is within their large receptive fields. The neurons are also largely oblivious to the lighting conditions or the distance of the object from the eye. These neurons have exactly the characteristics that are needed to identify a particular object across a wide range of viewing conditions—the kind of neurons that one would expect to see in a pathway specialized for perception.

The next important development was in the mid-1970s, when scientists began to record from visual neurons in the dorsal stream. This research had to await the development of techniques to record neurons while the monkey was awake and capable of moving its eyes and limbs. Working independently, Vernon Mountcastle at Johns Hopkins University, USA, and Juhani Hyvärinen in Helsinki, Finland, were the first to use these new methods to explore the properties of dorsal-stream neurons in detail. The surprising thing about many of these neurons is the fact that although they are visually responsive, most of them fire strongly only when the monkey actually responds in some way to the visual target. For example, some neurons fire only when the monkey reaches out toward a target; others require that the monkey flick their eyes (i.e. make "saccades") toward a stationary target; and still others fire to a moving target but only if the monkey follows it with its eyes. A particularly fascinating group of neurons, which were studied in detail during the 1990s by Hideo Sakata and his colleagues in Tokyo, Japan, respond when the monkey grasps or manipulates an object of a particular shape and orientation (see Figure 4.9).

These different subsets of neurons are clustered in somewhat separate areas of the posterior parietal cortex, clustered mostly along a prominent "sulcus" (literally a "groove" in Latin) in this region, known as the intraparietal sulcus (see Figure 4.10). The "grasp neurons," for example, are located mostly toward the front end of this sulcus in an area called the anterior intraparietal area (AIP). Lying right behind the AIP is the lateral intraparietal area (LIP), which contains neurons that fire when the monkey makes an eye movement to a visual stimulus (or even when it shifts its focus of attention to the stimulus without moving its eyes). And even further back, towards the boundary between the parietal and occipital lobes, there is a region known as area V6A, where the neurons fire in association with reaching movements of the arm and some aspects of grasping. But despite their differences, what most of the neurons in the dorsal stream have in common is that they do not fire unless

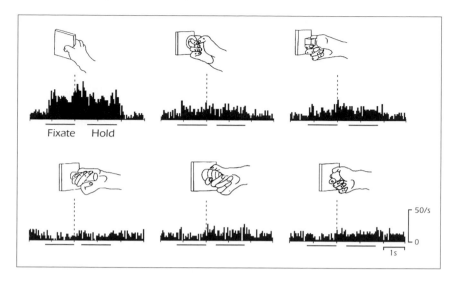

Figure 4.9 The activity of a neuron in area AIP when a monkey looks at and then grasps six different kinds of solid shapes. As the graphs below each shape show, this particular neuron responds best when the monkey grasps a vertically-oriented square plate. The neuron begins to fire when the monkey is first shown the object (marked "fixate") and continues to fire after the monkey has grasped it (marked "hold"). Other AIP neurons show similar patterns of activity but are tuned to quite different shapes and grasp postures. Reproduced from *Journal of Neurophysiology*, *83*(5), Selectivity for the shape, size, and orientation of objects for grasping in neurons of monkey parietal area AIP, Akira Murata, Vittorio Gallese, Giuseppe Luppino, Masakazu Kaseda, Hideo Sakata, 2000, 2580–2601, Figure 4, ©The American Physiological Society.

the monkey not only sees an object but in some way acts upon it as well. These are just the sorts of neurons you would expect to see in a "vision for action" pathway. Unlike the ventral stream, many dorsal-stream areas receive as much information from the visual periphery as they do from the central part of the retina. Some areas, like V6A, show a clear preference for objects presented in the lower part of the visual field. This makes perfect sense for structures involved in the visual control of action. When we reach out to grasp an object, for example, we not only have to process information about the object itself, we also have to monitor our moving limb, and avoid potential obstacles, both of which would typically lie well outside central vision and largely in the lower visual field.

Where do the two pathways lead to?

The evidence reviewed in this chapter suggests that the ventral stream of visual processing in the monkey is the main conduit for transforming visual signals into

73

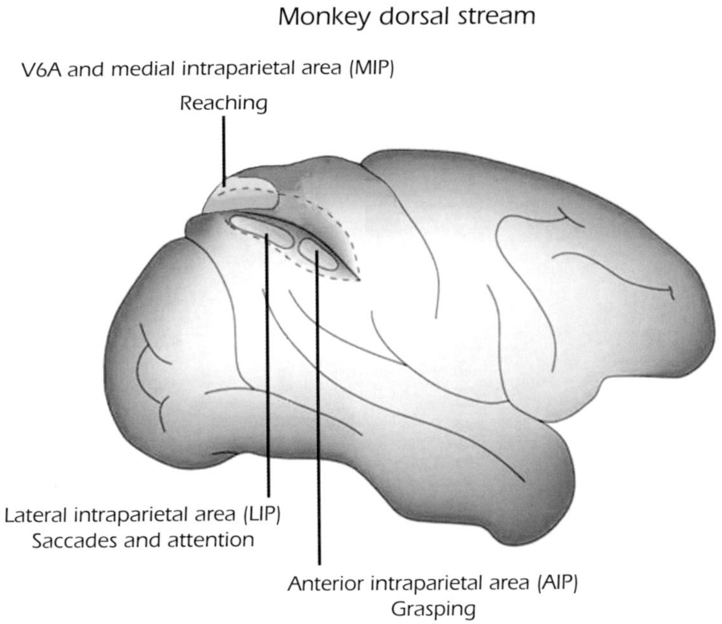

Monkey dorsal stream

Figure 4.10 Schematic diagram of the right hemisphere of the monkey's brain, showing the approximate locations of areas within the intraparietal sulcus (IPS) associated with visually guided movements of the eye, arm, and hand. Adapted by permission from Macmillan Publishers Ltd: Nature Reviews Neuroscience, 3 (7), pp. 553–562, (Figure 1), Yale E. Cohen and Richard A. Andersen, A common reference frame for movement plans in the posterior parietal cortex, © 2002.

perception whereas the dorsal stream plays the critical role in transforming visual signals into action (but see Box 4.4 for a discussion of a special sub-set of visuomotor neurons that appear to get input from the ventral stream as well). Not surprisingly, therefore, this division of labor is also reflected in the outputs of the two visual pathways.

BOX 4.4 MIRROR NEURONS

In the early 1990s, Giacomo Rizzolatti, a physiologist working in the University of Parma, Italy, made an astonishing discovery. For many years, Rizzolatti and his group had been recording the activity of single neurons in higher-order motor areas of the monkey brain, trying to work out how the firing of different neurons was related to the monkey's grasping movements as it reached out to pick up pieces of food. On one particular day, Rizzolatti was recording the activity of a neuron in the ventral premotor area (PMv), a brain region in the frontal lobes just in front of the primary motor cortex. So far, nothing seemed out of the ordinary. The firing

(Continued)

of the neuron was closely associated with the monkey's grasping movements, just like all the other neurons in this region that he and his research group had studied in the past. But then he noticed something quite remarkable. One of his young associates, who was standing in front of the monkey, began to pick up some of the peanuts that were scattered on the lab table. As he did so, the neuron in the monkey's brain continued to fire—but this time the firing was closely locked to the *associate's* grasping movements. Incredibly, Rizzolatti had found a neuron that fired not only when the monkey performed a particular action but also when the monkey observed another individual, even a member of another species, performing the same action (see box figure). Rizzolatti dubbed these cells "mirror neurons."

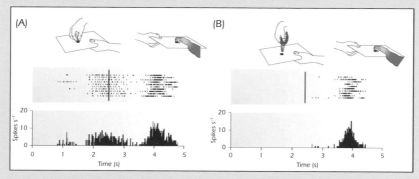

The activity of a mirror neuron recorded in the monkey PMv. (A) The successive traces in the top part of the figure show the neuron's responses while the monkey first observes a grasping movement made by the experimenter and then a short time later performs a similar grasping movement itself. The vertical line shows the time at which the experimenter's grasp is completed. (B) Here the piece of food is first grasped with pliers by the experimenter and then by the monkey. In this case the neuron fails to respond to the sight of the experimenter using pliers, but only when the monkey itself makes a grasp. Reproduced from *Nature Reviews Neuroscience*, 2, Neurophysiological mechanisms underlying the understanding and imitation of action, Giacomo Rizzolatti, Leonardo Fogassi, and Vittorio Gallese, 2001, 661–670 (figure1).

Since their discovery nearly twenty years ago, mirror neurons have been invoked to explain almost everything from action recognition to empathy. The central idea of what is sometimes called the "mirror neuron hypothesis" is that if the same neurons are driven both by performing an action and by observing another perform the same action then that "resonance" between action and action observation enables one to recognize the observed action through internal "simulation" rather than conceptual reasoning. But of course mirror neurons cannot do this all by themselves. After all, in order for the mirror neuron to "recognize" the action of picking up a piece of food, the neuron has to receive highly processed input from perceptual networks in and beyond the ventral stream that have analyzed the scene. These networks would have to extract form and motion information, match this to stored templates about what hands look like, and finally combine this with information about the goal and the spatial relationship between the hand and the goal. As it turns out, the ventral premotor area, where mirror neurons were first discovered, is part of a circuit that includes a higher-order ventral-stream area in the temporal lobe containing neurons that fire when the monkey views the actions

(Continued)

of others. These neurons, which were first described many years ago by our St Andrews colleague David Perrett, are not mirror neurons; they do not fire when the monkey itself makes an action—but they could provide the critical visual input that transforms ordinary grasping neurons into mirror neurons.

No matter where the visual input comes from, it seems pretty clear that a great deal of pre-processing has to be done to provide the mirror neuron with the visual input that resonates with the motor output that the neuron also codes. But if all that work has already been done, what extra information is provided by the firing of mirror neurons? The answer that some advocates of the mirror neuron hypothesis might give is that the recruitment of mirror neurons takes things beyond mere action recognition into the realm of action understanding; in other words, mirror neurons help the monkey to understand the actor's *intentions*. Indeed, some have argued that mirror neurons provided the evolutionary springboard for the emergence of complex social behavior, language, and culture in hominids.

But others have suggested that the mirror neuron hypothesis has been over-extended. The French philosopher Pierre Jacob, for example, has argued that the role of mirror neurons is not to compute the observed actor's goal or intention, but to compute instead the motor commands that the actor uses to achieve his or her goals. In other words, mirror neurons may be part of a system that computes the required actions to achieve a goal, working backwards from the perceived goal of the actor to generate a model (in the observer's brain) of the motor commands necessary to achieve that goal. Simply put, according to Jacob, mirror neurons may use information about intentions to code the required actions, not vice versa.

Whatever the function(s) of mirror neurons might be, there is no denying that their discovery has led to several promising lines of research—and has engaged the attention of psychologists and philosophers of mind. But one shouldn't be misled into thinking that the undeniably clear correspondence in firing for both action and action observation necessarily means that these neurons play a pivotal role in action understanding. Equally critical coding is almost certainly taking place in other neurons in the complex networks of which mirror neurons are a part—but the pattern of firing in the other neurons is much harder to map onto what is happening out in the world. The discovery of mirror neurons represents only the beginning of what is likely to be a complex account of how humans and other primates recognize and understand the actions of others.

REFERENCES

The following two books give a good flavor of this research and the different theoretical ideas to which it has led:

Iacoboni, M. (2009). *Mirroring people: The science of empathy and how we connect with others.* New York: Picador.

Rizzolatti, G. and Sinigaglia, C. (2007). *Mirrors in the Brain: How our minds share actions, emotions, and experience* (translated by F. Anderson). Oxford: Oxford University Press.

Consider the dorsal stream first. As we mentioned earlier, the behavioral repertoire of primates is much broader than that of the frog or even the gerbil. Fine hand and finger movements in particular imposed new demands on the visual system, and the evolutionary development of the dorsal stream can be seen as a response to these demands. It is no accident that the visuomotor areas in the posterior parietal cortex sit right next to the cortical areas that get tactile information from the hand and arm. These visuomotor areas are also intimately linked with parts of the motor cortex in the frontal lobe that send commands to the lower parts of the brain and the spinal cord. In fact, there are also direct pathways from the dorsal stream to lower parts of the brain, such as the superior colliculus, and to other way-stations that send instructions to the eye muscles and to parts of the spinal cord that control the limbs.

The ventral stream has none of these direct connections with motor systems. Instead, as befitting its role in perception and recognition, it interfaces with structures in the temporal and frontal lobes that have been implicated in memory, emotion, and social behavior. It is especially interesting, in the light of what we said earlier about the role of memory in perception, that these connections are very much two-way. Yet ultimately the perceptual system has to influence behavior. If it didn't, then it would never have evolved. The difference from the dorsal stream is that the ventral stream connections with the motor systems producing the behavior are much less direct. In fact, the connections can never be fully specified since the range of behavior that perception can influence is essentially infinite.

Summary

Vision serves behavior, but it does so in a variety of direct and indirect ways. What we can learn from studying other animals than ourselves is that there is not just one way of seeing, because we see for so many different purposes. Just as there is no sense in asking what David Ingle's frogs "see," it is important to realize that in many contexts it will make no sense to ask ourselves the same question. We are aware of what *one* of our visual systems tells us about the world, because we directly experience its products—our percepts of the world. But these experiences are not all there is to vision; there is a whole realm of visual processing, one that is primarily concerned with the control of our actions, which we can never experience or reflect on. We are certainly aware of the *movements* we make under the control of these systems, but we have no direct experience of the visual information these systems use.

Further Reading

The late David Ingle provided a compelling demonstration of the existence of parallel but independent visuomotor systems in a lower vertebrate in the following paper:

Ingle, D. (1973). Two visual systems in the frog. *Science, 181,* 1053–1055.

The evolution of brains is discussed (and beautifully illustrated) in the following book:

Allman, J.M. (1999). *Evolving Brains.* New York, NY: Scientific American Library.

This book by Semir Zeki provides a wonderful, if idiosyncratic, account of the physiology and anatomy of the primate visual system:

Zeki, S. (1993). *A Vision of the Brain.* Oxford: Blackwell Scientific Publications.

The following articles provide more detailed accounts of classic work on the monkey ventral and dorsal streams, respectively:

Andersen, R.A. and Buneo, C.A. (2003). Sensorimotor integration in posterior parietal cortex. *Advances in Neurology, 93,* 159–177.

Sakata, H., and Taira, M. (1994). Parietal control of hand action. *Current Opinion in Neurobiology, 4,* 847–856.

Tanaka, K. (1996). Inferotemporal cortex and object vision. *Annual Review of Neuroscience, 19,* 109–139.

For a detailed account of the division of labor between the dorsal and ventral streams, readers might wish to consult our earlier book, now in a second edition:

Milner, A.D. and Goodale, M.A. (2006). *The Visual Brain In Action* (2nd edition). Oxford: Oxford University Press.

This more recent article presents a detailed description and clarification of our theoretical model:

Milner, A.D. and Goodale, M.A. (2008). Two visual systems re-viewed. *Neuropsychologia, 46,* 774–785.

V

Streams within streams

Dee Fletcher is not blind, in any conventional sense of the word. For one thing, as we have emphasized already, she can use unconscious visual information to move around the world and interact with objects quite well. But in addition to this, many aspects of her conscious vision are also preserved. Dee continues to enjoy vivid and distinct experiences of color, for example, and can appreciate the fine detail of the surfaces of objects. This allows her still to take pleasure in looking at—and often correctly identifying—the blossoms and foliage of different plants and trees as she walks through her garden or is driven through the countryside. Dee's use of color contrasts sharply with her inability to recognize objects on the basis of their shape alone, for example, when shown black and white drawings of objects. She does a great deal better at identifying objects when their color or visual texture is present as well, as in a color photograph.

We saw in Chapter 2 (Box 2.1) that behavioral observations support the idea of separate visuomotor "channels" within the human dorsal stream, one for directing the hand in space and another for tailoring the hand grip to a particular target object. Dee's selective visual agnosia for shape argues for a multiplicity of channels in the domain of conscious perception as well, channels that need not all be damaged at once. In this chapter we will discuss more fully the evidence for such distinct visual modules in the human brain, within both the ventral and the dorsal streams.

How brain damage can affect our perception

The incomplete visual world that Dee lives in strongly suggests that the parts of the brain that are responsible for delivering our experiences of color and of form are different and separate from each other—and that only the part that deals with form perception has been damaged in her case. If so, then it would be expected that brain damage could occasionally cause the opposite pattern, causing a loss of color experience with a retained ability to recognize and distinguish different shapes.

As it turns out, this pattern of visual loss does sometimes occur. Individuals with this problem, known as "cerebral achromatopsia," have a special form of color blindness in which the color-sensitive cones in the eye are all working normally but the apparatus in the brain that provides the experience of color is damaged. Yet strange as it may seem, individuals who have developed achromatopsia are often able to see the borders between two equally bright colors, say red and green, even though they are completely unable to say which side is red and which side is green (see Figure 5.1). Achromatopsia is not a color-naming problem. An individual with achromatopsia can tell you that bananas are yellow, yet when asked to color in a line drawing of a banana is just as likely to use the blue or red crayon as the yellow one. They sometimes describe seeing the world in various shades of gray. Dee has at least been spared this understandably depressing kind of experience, which is described graphically in Oliver Sacks's essay "The case of the color-blind painter" in his well-known book *An Anthropologist on Mars*.

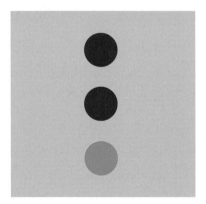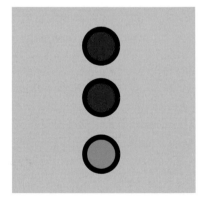

Figure 5.1 Martin Smithson, who has achromatopsia, cannot see colors but can see the boundaries between areas of different colors. Thus, he can tell the odd man out in the display on the left, where there are color boundaries, but he cannot tell the three disks apart when those boundaries are covered over by black lines, as on the right. Reprinted from *Neuropsychologia*, *42*(6), R.W. Kentridge, C.A. Heywood, and A. Cowey, Chromatic edges, surfaces and constancies in cerebral achromatopsia, pp. 821–830, © (2004), with permission from Elsevier.

Charles Heywood and his colleagues have carried out extensive studies of the color vision of an achromatopsic patient we will call Martin Smithson, who suffered brain damage while serving as a young police cadet. Like Dee, Martin has visual agnosia, but he shows the exact opposite pattern from her when it comes to colors and shapes. While Dee can distinguish colors but not shapes, Martin can distinguish shapes but not colors. Interestingly, telling apart different visual textures (imagine the difference between seeing a fragment of fur and a fragment of woven cloth of identical plain color) seems to be closely associated with color discrimination in the brain. Thus Dee can distinguish textures well, but Martin is quite unable to tell one from another.

These contrasts between Dee's and Martin's visual experience provide further examples of "double dissociation," an idea that we introduced in Chapter 3. In that chapter, however, we were making a distinction between two broad categories of visual processing—one devoted to delivering our perceptions, the other to guiding our actions. We noted that each of those functions could be separately and independently disrupted by brain damage, in the ventral stream in the case of perception, or the dorsal stream in the case of action. But what we are seeing in Dee and Martin is that even within one of those streams, the ventral stream, there are double dissociations as well. Not surprisingly, as we shall see later, Dee and Martin have damage to slightly different parts of the ventral stream—with each region being responsible for processing different features of the visual world. So what does this mean for everyday perception? You may think that you see a single integrated representation of a visual scene, like an image on a movie screen, but the evidence from Dee and Martin strongly suggests that your brain is actually analyzing different aspects of the scene separately using different visual modules. The products of these modules may never be combined into a single "picture" in the brain—though they clearly have to be cross-referenced or bound together in some way. After all, the brain has to be able to distinguish between a red pepper on a green plate and a green pepper on a red plate.

Of course colors, textures, and shapes are basic and ubiquitous features of our visual experience, features that we use to distinguish among different instances of the things we know in everyday life—such as different man-made objects, animals, plants, major landmarks, or other people. These features are essentially about the physics of the objects—their three-dimensional geometry or macrostructure on the one hand, and their surface microstructure (color, glossiness, texture) on the other. But at a higher level of analysis, we need to be able to categorize what sorts of objects we are looking at. Is this conglomerate of visual features an animal, a tool, a face, a person, or something else? The evidence from clinical neurology strongly suggests that damage to different areas within the ventral stream can result in deficits in recognition that appear to be limited to one category of things in the world and not others.

Perhaps the best-known example of this is the condition known as "prosopagnosia" (from the Greek *prosopon*, meaning person). An individual who suffers from this problem may be quite unable to recognize even a close member of their family, or a famous personality, when all they have to go on is the person's face. They generally have no difficulty when they hear the person speak, or even when they see the person moving around in habitual ways. Of course there are many aspects of a face that our brains take into account when we recognize a person: skin coloration and texture, hair color and hairline, facial shape, and the placement of features like the eyes and mouth. Nonetheless, it is striking that a person with prosopagnosia typically does not have a general agnosia for objects. It is just faces they have a problem with.

For example, the neuropsychologist Bruno Rossion has carried out a number of studies of a Belgian woman, Paule Soulier, who suffered a severe head injury while on a visit to England. Unaccustomed to traffic driving on the left, she looked the wrong way when stepping out to cross a busy street in London, and was hit head-on by a bus. Although Mme Soulier recovered remarkably well, she was left with a profound prosopagnosia, for example, being quite unable to recognize the faces of famous people such as movie stars, people whose faces had been very familiar to her before her accident. Yet she had no difficulty in perceiving and identifying different inanimate objects.

Perhaps more remarkably, a study by Morris Moscovitch and his colleagues in Toronto, Canada, documented the case of a man, Charles K., whose brain damage has caused the opposite pattern—a devastating loss in the ability to recognize objects without any problem in recognizing faces (see Figures 5.2 and 5.3). This fascinating case provides us with yet another double dissociation: "faces lost, objects intact" in one person, "faces intact, objects lost" in the other.

So the clinical evidence suggests that there is modularity in the ventral stream on at least two levels. We see it first at the level of primitive visual features (color, edges, motion), which are each processed by quite separate systems. But these modules do not then simply join together to feed into a general-purpose visual recognition system. Rather, these lower-level channels evidently feed their information into multiple higher-level systems, each specialized for a particular category of things in the world.

Faces undoubtedly constitute a unique visual category for human beings, and for good reason. The recognition of individuals plays a critical role in everyday interactions in social animals like monkeys and humans, and an ability to identify faces is a highly reliable way to achieve this. So important are faces in our daily lives that we often imagine that we see them in places where they don't exist, for example, on

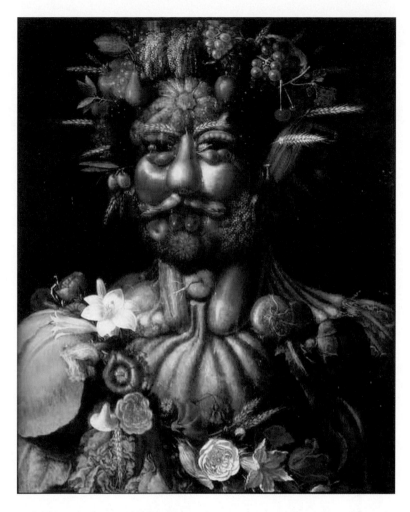

Figure 5.2 This painting, entitled *Verdumnus*, is one of a series by Italian painter, Giuseppe Arcimbaldo (1530–1593), that depict faces constructed of other objects, in this case fruits and vegetables. When the object agnosia patient, Charles K., looked at this painting, he saw the face right away but failed to identify any of the fruits and vegetables that make up the face.

the surface of the moon. Notably, the identification of faces takes place in a rapid, holistic way rather than in a feature-by-feature fashion. Thus, for example, we can detect family resemblances between individuals without being able to point to how we do it. (For two other examples of the specialized nature of face recognition, see Figures 5.4 and 5.5).

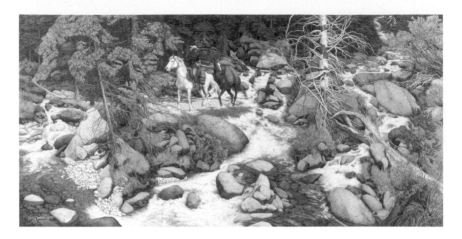

Figure 5.3 This painting by the American artist, Bev Doolittle, *The Forest Has Eyes*, conceals a number of faces hidden in the trees and rocks. Whereas the face in the Arcimbaldo painting is immediately obvious, the faces here are much more difficult to see. But Charles K. spotted them immediately—and was not confused by the other elements of the painting, which to the normal observer are far more salient. The Forest Has Eyes © Bev Doolittle, licensed by The Greenwich Workshop, Inc.

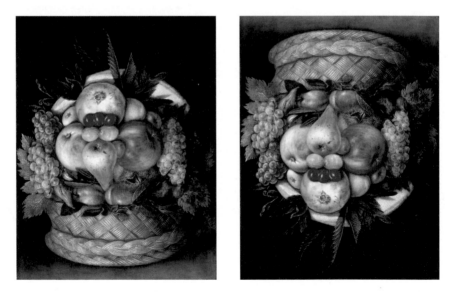

Figure 5.4 Arcimbaldo was a surrealist—centuries before the term was invented. This painting, *Reversible Head with Basket of Fruit*, is one of several which create totally different perceptual images when inverted. It shows very clearly how our perception of faces depends critically on the orientation of the image.

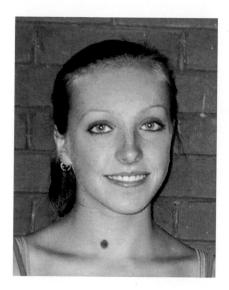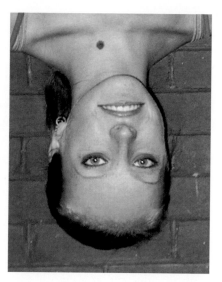

Figure 5.5 These two photographs of a young woman illustrate the specialized nature of face process-ing, in which the normal upright face is treated as a whole rather than as a collection of separate features. If you turn the page upside down, your face processing module will immediately allow you to see that there is something dreadfully wrong with one of pictures! When viewing the page the right way up, the face on the right looks relatively normal because upside-down faces do not engage the "holistic" face processing module and instead the brain has to deal with each feature separately.

But faces are not the only category of special objects that have their own dedicated hardware in the brain that when damaged can cause a specific agnosia. Another, less well-known, example of this is where a person loses the ability to find their way around a once-familiar environment, such as their hometown. This so-called "topographical agnosia" can in many cases be attributed to a loss of recognition for particular major landmarks, such as a street corner church or store. We generally use landmarks of these kinds in orienting ourselves and in constructing an internal map of our environment. Topographical agnosia was first described by the pioneer-ing English neurologist John Hughlings Jackson in 1876. Jackson was actually the first person to recognize the existence of visual agnosia (though he called it "imper-ception" rather than agnosia). His patient suffered from prosopagnosia as well as topographical agnosia, a co-occurrence that turns out to be quite frequent. But each can occur without the other, suggesting that their co-occurrence is simply due to the accidental damage of two quite differently specialized mechanisms that may per-haps lie close together in the brain. In fact only a minority of agnosic patients have their recognition difficulties restricted to a single domain, as in prosopagnosia or topographical agnosia. Dee Fletcher, for example, is herself prosopagnosic, in addition to having a severe object agnosia.

Seeing inside the brain

These inferences from clinical observations have been reinforced in recent years by a number of functional brain imaging studies, in which healthy people view pictures of objects of different kinds, while the activation pattern in their brains (generally as inferred from the changes in blood flow through the vessels that supply the brain) is measured (see Box 5.1). Brain imaging not only allows us to "look inside the heads" of brain-damaged people to find out where their damage is located, but also to eavesdrop inside the heads of *un*damaged individuals to map which areas change their activity when the person sees or does particular things. For example, Semir Zeki and his collaborators in University College London, UK, discovered over twenty years ago that an abstract Mondrian-style pattern made up of different-colored patches activates a different set of cortical areas than a comparable pattern composed only of different shades of gray. When the two activation maps were subtracted from each other, a particular part of the brain could be seen to be selectively associated with viewing the colored pattern. Gratifyingly, this "color area" corresponds closely to the area where damage causes achromatopsia.

BOX 5.1 FUNCTIONAL NEUROIMAGING

The development of new imaging techniques has enabled scientists to pinpoint the activity of different regions of the brain with considerable accuracy. Positron emission tomography (PET) scanning, the technique of choice up until the late 1990s, is now rarely used in research with human subjects, partly because it involves the injection of radioactive isotopes into the bloodstream. Currently the most widely used technique is functional magnetic resonance imaging (fMRI), which has a much higher spatial resolution, of up to 1 mm^3 or better, and does not require any invasive procedure. In fact, because it is so safe, people can be scanned many times. FMRI is an adaptation of an earlier technique called magnetic resonance imaging (or MRI) in which the three-dimensional structure of the brain can be visualized using high magnetic fields.

To make an MRI of the brain, the person's head is placed inside a strong magnetic field (sometimes more than 100,000 times more powerful than the earth's magnetic field). The hydrogen atoms in the various molecules in the person's brain tissue align with that magnetic field (a bit like a compass needle aligning with the earth's magnetic field). A short pulse of radiofrequency energy is then administered to the brain causing the alignment of the hydrogen atoms to be perturbed. As the atoms return to their original alignment in the magnetic field, they give off tiny amounts of energy that can be detected by an antenna or "receiver" coil placed around the head. Because the density of water (and thus hydrogen

(Continued)

atoms) varies systematically between the gray and white matter of the brain (i.e. between the cell bodies and the connecting fibers), the three-dimensional anatomical structure of the brain can be reconstructed based on the differences in the strength of the signals generated by different kinds of brain tissue.

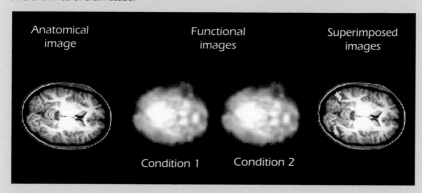

The subtraction logic frequently used in functional neuro-imaging research is shown in the figure. Scans of the activity patterns in the brain in the experimental condition (say, viewing intact line drawings of objects—"condition 1") are compared with scans derived from a control condition (say, viewing fragmented versions of the same drawings—"condition 2"). The difference (shown on the right) represents the areas specifically activated by object drawings, "partialling out" more basic visual processing. Conventionally "false colors" are used in producing these difference maps, showing the "hottest" areas in yellow, the less hot in red, and so on. These colored areas are superimposed on an anatomical MRI image of the brain of the same individual. All of the scans shown here represent a horizontal cross-section through the brain at the level of the temporal lobe.

FMRI exploits the fact that oxygenated blood has different magnetic properties from deoxygenated blood. Hydrogen atoms that are in the vicinity of oxygenated blood in active brain areas give off a slightly different signal from hydrogen molecules near deoxygenated blood. The receiver coil picks up the blood oxygen-level dependent (BOLD) signals, which reflect increased activity of neurons in particular brain areas. The BOLD signals measured when a person performs one task in the magnet can be compared to the BOLD signals that are measured when the person performs another task. The difference between these BOLD signals can then be mapped onto a detailed structural MRI of the brain—revealing patterns of activity that are correlated with the performance of one kind of task but not another.

Techniques have also been developed that can harness fMRI to provide three-dimensional maps of major fiber tracts, the bundles of nerve fibers connecting one brain area with another. One of these techniques, known as diffusion tensor imaging (DTI), depends on the fact that water diffuses more rapidly along the length of the fiber tract, and more slowly in directions perpendicular to the tract. Because the rate of diffusion affects the MRI signal, one can get an idea of the route that a fiber tract follows. Note, however, that DTI doesn't reveal which direction the information is flowing along that tract.

Color, of course, is just one of several "surface features" that an object can have, along with its texture, brightness, glossiness, and detailed surface pattern. These various surface features can characterize different kinds of material (wood, plastic, fur, cloth, etc.), and so can help us to identify what "stuff" a given object is made of (see Figure 5.6). It turns out from functional magnetic resonance imaging (fMRI) studies (see Box 5.1) with healthy volunteers that these other surface features activate brain areas right next to and overlapping with the "color areas" (see Figure 5.7), so it is perhaps not surprising that Dee, whose color vision has survived her brain damage, has also retained an acute awareness of these other surface properties of objects. Conversely the proximity of these areas explains why our achromatopsic patient Martin Smithson, who has lost his "color" areas, has also lost his ability to distinguish different visual textures. Here again then, studies of brain damaged patients mesh neatly with modern neuroimaging research to help us understand the workings of the modules or "channels" of visual processing that ultimately lead to our integrated perception of everyday objects.

Similar functional imaging studies have confirmed the existence of separate areas dedicated respectively to the perception of faces and places. For example, Nancy

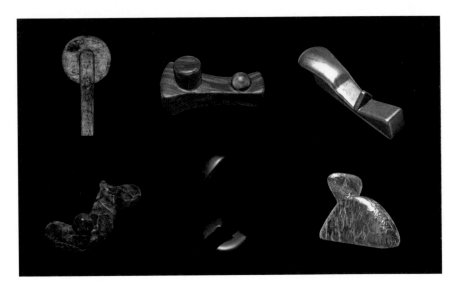

Figure 5.6 These artificial "objects," in which shape and surface properties can be separately varied, are examples of images that were used in a series of fMRI experiments carried by our colleague, Jon Cant, to investigate the brain areas involved in processing different features of objects (see Figure 5.7). Reprinted from Jonathan S. Cant and Melvyn A. Goodale, Attention to form or surface properties modulates different regions of human occipitotemporal cortex, *Cerebral Cortex*, 2007, *17*(3), 713–731, Figure 1, with permission from Oxford University Press.

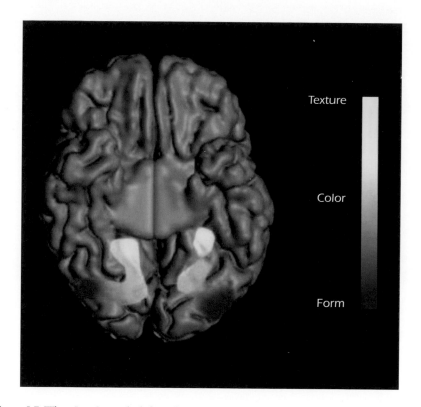

Figure 5.7 When Jon Cant asked the volunteers in his experiment to attend to the shape of the images as shown in Figure 5.6, areas shown in red on the lateral part of the ventral occipital cortex were activated, but when they were asked to attend to the color or surface texture of the objects, more medial areas, shown in orange and yellow, were activated. As can be seen, the areas responsive to color and texture overlapped quite a bit. Reprinted from *Trends in Cognitive Sciences*, 13(7), Eagleman, David M., and Goodale, Melvyn A., Why color synesthesia involves more than color, pp. 288–292, Figure 2. © (2009), with permission from Elsevier.

Kanwisher at MIT, USA, has identified a "face area" in a part of the ventral stream called the fusiform cortex. This area, which she named FFA (fusiform face area), is activated much more by pictures of faces than by pictures of other everyday objects, buildings, or even scrambled pictures of faces (see Figure 5.8 right). We now know that there are at least two other areas specialized for face perception. One is located in the occipital lobe (see Figure 5.8 left) and is referred to as the occipital face area (OFA) and appears to play a role in the early processing of faces; another, buried in the superior temporal sulcus, is involved in processing facial movements and emotional expressions. (Interestingly, even though Dee can often tell the difference between a face and an inanimate object, she can't recognize individual faces or

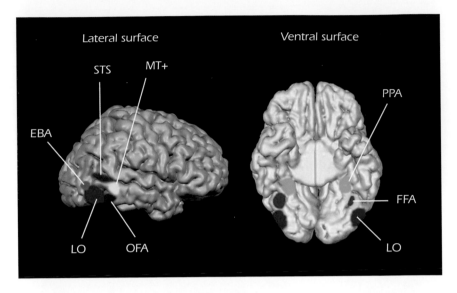

Figure 5.8 Lateral and ventral views of the right hemisphere of the human brain showing the location of visual areas apparently specialized for different categories and features of objects. These include the lateral occipital area (LO), the fusiform face area (FFA), the parahippocampal place area (PPA), the extrastriate body area (EBA), the occipital face area (OFA), part of the superior temporal sulcus (STS), and the human motion area (MT+).

detect differences in facial expression. The reason for this appears not to be related to damage in FFA, which is spared, but rather to the fact that her brain damage includes area OFA on both sides.)

These face-specific areas are separate from another area in the ventral stream, the parahippocampal place area or PPA, which is activated by pictures of buildings and scenes, but much less by pictures of faces or pictures of tools or other small objects (Figure 5.8 right). Russell Epstein, a neuroscientist now based in the University of Pennsylvania, was one of the first to identify the PPA and to show that this ventral—stream area was particularly sensitive to the appearance and layout of scenes. As he and others have pointed out, damage to this region is typically associated with topographical agnosia, which, as we saw earlier, is a deficit in finding one's way around familiar environments.

Yet another area has been identified which relates to the shapes that define everyday objects (like fruit, cups, TV sets, and vases). This region, generally called the lateral occipital area (or area LO) is revealed by taking fMRI scans while people look either at pictures of intact objects or at scrambled pictures of objects and then subtracting the two scan images (see Figure 5.8 right). This subtraction removes the brain activation caused just by the constituent lines and edges, leaving behind the activity related specifically to the structure present in the intact pictures (see Box 5.1). As we saw earlier, this same area was activated when people were asked to concentrate on the shape of an object rather than on its color or texture (see Figures 5.6 and 5.7). These kinds of experiments have led to the idea that area LO is specialized for analyzing the geometrical structure of objects. As we shall see later in this chapter, this particular area is very important for understanding Dee's perceptual problems.

The number of specialized areas that have been identified within the human ventral stream continues to grow. For example, we now know there are areas that are more responsive to images of human body parts than they are to faces. One such "body area" (the extrastriate body area or EBA) is located close to areas LO, while another (the fusiform body area or FBA) lies immediately adjacent to the FFA. In other work, Cristiana Cavina-Pratesi, Magdalena Ietswaart, and their colleagues in Durham and Newcastle in the UK have recently discovered a "hand area" adjacent to the left EBA, which responds strongly to human hands (and to a lesser extent to robotic hands, fingers, and feet) but not at all to other body parts.

The critical areas for all these different visual categories are located close together on the underside of the brain around the junction of the occipital and temporal lobes (see Figure 5.8). Although the degree of overlap among the different areas remains controversial, there is no doubting their separate existence and relative specialization. Thus the brain imaging experiments and the clinical studies both point to one undeniable conclusion: our perceptual experience is not the product of a general purpose object recognition system but is instead the creation of a set of quasi-independent visual modules (see Box 5.2 for an example of how movies can be used together with brain imaging to demonstrate the activation of different brain areas by different classes of visual stimuli). There is some debate, however, about whether the areas associated with the recognition of particular categories of visual stimuli (faces, places, and objects, for example), are really dedicated to those precise categories—or instead happen to be regions in the ventral stream that process the right combination of features that are essential for recognizing one category rather than another.

BOX 5.2 WATCHING MOVIES IN THE SCANNER

One of the perennially intriguing questions in psychology and philosophy is whether two different people looking at the same events at the same time truly experience them in the same way. We don't have the technology yet to scan people's brain activity as they live their everyday lives, but we can show people the same movie in the fMRI scanner and compare how their brains react to it. Rafi Malach and colleagues, at the Weizmann Institute of Science in

(Continued)

91

Israel, had each of their volunteers watch a segment of the Clint Eastwood movie *The Good, the Bad, and the Ugly* while lying in the scanner. They then tested whether or not the fMRI activations from one person's brain could be used to predict the activation patterns in another person's brain as that second person watched the same movie. Remarkably, they found they could successfully predict the fMRI activation patterns across about 25–30 percent of the surface area of the other brain.

Two kinds of brain areas showed these inter-brain correlations most clearly. First, perhaps not surprisingly, regions linked to emotional reactions behaved in a similar way across the different viewers during scenes in the film that were emotionally arousing. But more relevantly for the present discussion, this was also true for areas selective for visual categories like faces and places. So the FFA, the region that responds strongly to faces, showed similarly robust responses in different observers whenever faces appeared on the screen, especially during close-up shots of faces. Likewise, the PPA responded vigorously in all the viewers whenever the movie showed images of indoor and outdoor scenes, including buildings.

Of course the fact that not all brain activity matched up perfectly between different people should come as no surprise—we all bring different attitudes, preferences, and expectations with us when we visit the cinema (as in life), and take away with us different messages and interpretations of what we see. Such differences between people are presumably represented somewhere in that 70 percent or so of the brain's tissue that does not behave in a predictable way.

One of the most satisfying aspects of this research is that it shows we can generalize fMRI results from the highly artificial to what is (almost) real life. After all, in a typical fMRI experiment, the participants view a fixed sequence of strictly controlled images (usually stationary) and perform an arbitrary task such as pushing a button whenever an image is repeated. But here people could look wherever they liked at the screen in front of them, choosing freely what they wanted to look at and reacting internally in their own ways. Yet still the same areas like the FFA and PPA responded to faces and places respectively, showing the validity of the "artificial" fMRI studies that discovered these areas in the first place.

The movie experiment also breaks new ground in a different way—it reverses the logic of the typical fMRI experiment. In a traditional fMRI experiment, the participants are shown specific images of different kinds of objects (faces, places, and tools, for example) and then the scans of their brains are examined to see what areas are activated. In Malach's study, the different patterns of activation in the brains of several participants viewing the movie are intercorrelated to identify regions that are activated at the same point in the movie. Then the movie is examined to find out what image was present to cause this common activation. In other words, the investigators could now ask what visual stimulus caused a given activation rather than what activation was caused by a given visual stimulus.

REFERENCE

Hasson, U., Nir, Y., Levy, I., Fuhrmann, G., and Malach, R. (2004). Intersubject synchronization of cortical activity during natural vision. *Science, 303*, 1634–1640.

"Reversible lesions" in the human brain

Historically, studies of people with selective brain damage have been hugely important in forming hypotheses about what goes on where in the human brain, and when the results of later neuroimaging research agree with those hypotheses, as they usually do, they provide strong convergent support for them. But this works both ways: the results of neuroimaging alone are highly ambiguous without complementary support. After all, how do we know that activation of area X during a particular kind of behavior plays a causal role in determining that behavior, rather than just being an epiphenomenon, with the real causal processes going on somewhere else altogether? So studying brain-damaged individuals has by no means become redundant with the advent of sophisticated fMRI methodologies. On the other hand, however, there is no such thing as a person with damage to area X which is confined to area X, and which has destroyed all of area X. After all, damage to the human brain typically arises from head trauma, tumors, strokes, and, in some cases, degenerative diseases, none of which respect the boundaries between different functional areas. Experimental lesions in animals, of course, can achieve this, which is why animal research has been so valuable in the past. For obvious reasons such an approach is unacceptable in humans. Nonetheless, it would be useful if researchers could find a way to selectively disable area X in humans without disabling other areas. As it turns out, the technique of transcranial magnetic stimulation (TMS) comes close to doing that.

TMS (see Box 5.3) can temporarily disable a group of neurons in a normal healthy brain by over-stimulating them; they revert to normal shortly afterwards. In this way TMS can mimic the effects of real brain damage, albeit over a short timescale. This means that like real brain damage it can give us strong empirical evidence about cause and effect.

BOX 5.3 TRANSCRANIAL MAGNETIC STIMULATION (TMS)

TMS is a non-invasive procedure that can be used to cause temporary disruption of normal brain activity. Thus, TMS allows researchers to study the function of and interaction between brain areas in neurologically intact volunteers. TMS is administered by holding a plastic-enclosed coil of wire next to the head to create a rapidly changing magnetic field. This induces weak electric currents in the brain by means of electromagnetic induction, thereby causing the neurons lying immediately beneath the coil to fire in an abnormal manner (i.e. all at once). TMS causes minimal discomfort to the person receiving the stimulation, and in small doses has no detectable long-lasting effect on brain function.

(Continued)

The great merit of TMS is that it allows us to ask questions about the causal role of a particular brain area in a psychological or behavioral task of interest. According to whether or not task performance is impaired (or enhanced), we can determine whether the area is truly involved in the processing of a task or instead is merely co-activated when the task is performed.

Because the effects of a brief pulse of TMS are short-lasting, pulses delivered at specific times during the performance of a task such as visually guided grasping can provide a window into the timing of the underlying brain processes. Repeated long trains of TMS pulses can interfere with brain processing for some length of time afterwards (often several minutes) and thus can be used to 'knock out' a particular brain area for some time. Repetitive TMS of this kind can have long-term effects as well and has been used successfully to treat a number of medical conditions including migraines, tinnitus, depression, and auditory hallucinations.

TMS studies of many areas in the ventral stream such as the FFA and PPA are impossible to carry out because those structures lie on the underside of the cerebral hemispheres out of range of the TMS coil (which can stimulate brain tissue only a couple of centimeters below the skull). Other ventral stream areas, however, lie completely on the side of the occipital lobe, such as area EBA, and so can easily be accessed for TMS experiments. As we saw earlier, area EBA shows fMRI activations specifically when bodies or body parts are viewed. In one study, Salvatore Aglioti and his colleagues at the University of Verona found that applying TMS to the EBA caused a slowing of reaction times when people were required to discriminate quickly between different body parts, but not in tasks where they had to discriminate between different parts of the face or different components of motorcycles. TMS applied to other areas in the vicinity of the EBA had no such effect.

Motion vision: a special case

The cluster of visual areas on, or close to, the underside of the occipital and temporal lobes that we have been discussing so far seems to house most of the machinery that underlies our perceptual experience. But not all disorders of perception are linked to this brain region. One particular selective loss, sometimes known as *akinetopsia*, is associated with damage to a rather different part of the brain. In this very rare condition, the patient loses the ability to see motion. An individual with akinetopsia will be able to see stationary objects perfectly well, but will soon lose track of any object that is moving relatively quickly. For example, the neuropsychologist Josef Zihl described a patient living in Munich who had difficulty pouring coffee into a cup, because she could not see the level of the liquid rising—she saw it as a series of stationary snapshots instead. She sometimes experienced an everyday scene as being filled with jerky movements rather as if it were stroboscopically illuminated, or as if she were watching an old silent movie. Crossing the street was a nightmare for her. At one moment, a car would seem stationary some distance away, and the next moment it would seem to have jumped right in front of her. She literally never saw it coming.

Interestingly, while many cases have been described of patients whose brain damage has caused combinations of prosopagnosia, achromatopsia, and topographical agnosia, these disorders are hardly ever seen in combination with akinetopsia. The reason for this is more geographical than functional. As can be seen in the brain maps shown in Figure 5.8, the layout of the visual areas that deal with faces, colors, and places all lie in close proximity to each other on the underside of the brain, so that damage to one is quite likely to impinge on one or more of the other areas. In contrast, the "motion area" lies some way away, still within the temporal lobe, but up above area LO on the side of the brain. This motion area was first identified almost forty years ago in the monkey by Semir Zeki, who showed that it gets direct inputs from the primary visual cortex. Zeki went on to show that individual neurons in this area (which he called V5, though it is now usually called MT, since it lies near the middle of the temporal lobe) would fire only when a moving visual spot was shown to the monkey in a particular part of its visual field. Moreover, the spot not only had to be moving but had to be going in a certain direction at a certain speed. What did not matter, however, was the color, shape, or visual texture of the moving spot.

The motion area in humans was first identified using positron emission tomography (PET). The responses in this area are very similar to those observed in monkey MT—and for this reason the area in the human brain has been dubbed area MT+. Applying TMS to area MT+ reliably invokes "motion phosphenes," sensations of visual motion, typically experienced as moving spots of light. The production of such hallucinatory experiences of motion following stimulation of area MT+ shows that activity in this region (even abnormally produced activity) plays a causal role in our perception of motion.

By analyzing motion within the visual scene, area MT+ adds the "fourth dimension" to our perceptual life. This is crucial for us to be able to interpret and predict the movements of other people as well as other animals. In fact recent research has revealed yet more specialized areas that seem to piece together this kind of information about other people's behavior. As we saw earlier, there are brain areas that are particularly concerned with static views of the body or body parts. But there is another region, buried in the posterior part of the superior temporal sulcus close to the area specialized for processing facial movements mentioned earlier, that prefers bodies in motion. This area was first discovered in the monkey by David Perrett in St Andrews (see Chapter 4, Box 4.4), and has now been clearly identified in the human brain. The area even responds to the so-called "biological motion" movie clips originally devised by Gunnar Johansson in Uppsala, Sweden. In Johansson's displays, a few points of light moving on a screen give an irresistible impression of, for example, a man walking on the spot or a woman doing pirouettes. When a single frame of the movie is frozen, you may still be able to tell if it is a man or a woman but you would have little idea what the person is doing. He or she could be dancing, walking, running, or jumping. Only when the display is moving is the activity of the person unambiguously clear. What we are seeing in these higher reaches of the ventral stream is the brain machinery that adds the fourth dimension (motion) to the three dimensions of body form, providing the information we need to recognize and understand the behavior of other individuals.

Area MT is notably different from the other areas we have been discussing in that it does not clearly belong to one visual stream or the other. It is located "early" in the wiring diagram that links all of the areas back to the primary visual cortex V1, and sends its outputs not only toward the ventral-stream areas we have been discussing, but also to areas in the dorsal stream concerned with controlling action (see Chapter 4, Box 4.1).

The building blocks of visually guided action

Just as there is modularity in the human ventral stream, so there is also modularity in the human dorsal stream. But the modularity in the dorsal stream is based not on the particular visual elements that a given brain area deals with, so much as on the nature of the actions that are guided by those visual elements—just as we saw in the monkey, in Chapter 4. These actions include things like reaching, saccadic (quick) eye movements, pursuit (slow) eye movements, grasping with the hand, and whole-body locomotion. Of course these elementary actions rarely occur in isolation in everyday behavior. Instead, they are combined in an infinite number of different ways to serve our behavioral needs. For example, to pick up a coffee cup from the table, we might walk toward the table, move our eyes to look at the cup, extend our hand toward it without colliding with anything else on the table while simultaneously configuring the posture of fingers in readiness to grasp the cup's handle, and then finally grasp it and pick it up. These different action elements would never be put together in exactly the same way on two different occasions. In fact, each element would have to be individually guided by different visual information. So although there must be some kind of overall orchestration of the different elements of the action, each element also needs its own visual guidance system. It was this need for separate guidance systems that must have led to the evolution of separate visuomotor modules in the posterior parietal cortex, each of which is responsible for the visual control of a particular class of movements. There is also evidence that these visuomotor modules operate somewhat differently on the two sides of the brain (see Box 5.4).

BOX 5.4 THE ASYMMETRICAL BRAIN

One of the unique things about the human brain is its functional asymmetry. It *looks* pretty symmetrical, just as people themselves do—but like people, it *works* asymmetrically. Most readers will have come across the idea that the left hemisphere is verbal and "logical," while the right is visual and "creative." There is some truth to these notions, though the contrasts are not quite as clear-cut as the popular press would have us believe.

There is good evidence from neuropsychological studies of brain-damaged patients that visual recognition of familiar faces and places is mostly handled by the ventral stream in the right hemisphere. Prosopagnosia and topographical agnosia, for example, arise much more often from right ventral-stream lesions than from left. It's the same story in functional brain imaging studies: when people look at pictures of faces and places, there is typically more activation in the face and place areas of their right hemisphere than there is in the corresponding areas on the left. The reason why a good deal of ventral-stream processing is concentrated in the right hemisphere is not well understood. One possible explanation is that many of the corresponding areas in the left hemisphere are busy doing quite different jobs, particularly ones concerned with speech and language. It may be that language and perception depend on brain systems that operate on such different principles that they can't work in close proximity with each other.

In contrast, the early visual areas are quite symmetrically organized on the two sides of the brain, with the left side of the brain representing the right half of the visual field, and vice versa. In the same way, the motor cortex is symmetrically organized. People with strokes invading the motor cortex in the left hemisphere invariably show a right-side motor weakness or paralysis, and again vice versa. The fact that the early sensory systems and later motor control systems are completely symmetrical is no surprise. After all, these are the parts of the brain that interact directly with the outside world, which has no intrinsic left/right biases. They are organized this way in all vertebrates. Because the dorsal stream has the job of converting visual input into motor output, it would make sense if it too were symmetrically distributed across both hemispheres. It would not be efficient to have these visuomotor systems concentrated in one hemisphere, since we have to be able to respond to visual targets on our right and left equally well. As it turns out, however, things are not quite that simple. It is certainly true that most functional brain imaging studies of visuomotor control find dorsal-stream activations on the two sides of the brain to a roughly symmetrical extent. It is also true that patients with left or right parietal damage are equally likely to develop unilateral optic ataxia. This unilateral damage always causes misreaching, by either hand, when the target

(Continued)

97

lies in the visual field opposite the side of the damage. After left parietal damage, however, as Perenin and Vighetto discovered in the 1980s, an additional "hand effect" is often present, causing misreaching by the opposite (right) hand *wherever* the target is. This hand effect is rarely seen after right parietal damage.

These different visuomotor areas in the parietal cortex are linked with similarly dedicated regions within part of the frontal lobe known as the premotor cortex. In other words, the dorsal stream's modules are probably better described as parietofrontal modules. As mentioned in Chapter 4, these modules also link up with sensorimotor control structures (like the superior colliculus and cerebellum) in the lower, more ancient parts of the brain. These structures are dedicated to the production of elementary eye or limb movements whose output parameters are highly specified. As we suggested in Chapter 4, the newer parietofrontal modules can be regarded as constituting a high-level "managerial" system, which provides flexible control over these older and more "reflexive" visuomotor networks in the brainstem.

Just as was the case for the ventral stream, the evidence for separate and specialized dorsal-stream modules in humans came initially from clinical studies of patients with damage in localized regions of the cerebral cortex. The classic Bálint syndrome (exemplified by Ruth Vickers and Anne Thiérry: see Chapter 3) is characterized by a host of visuomotor disabilities, ranging from difficulties in making saccadic eye movements through to problems with visually guided reaching and grasping. Of course, in these patients the damaged areas are typically quite large, including most of the parietal lobe on both sides of the brain. Nevertheless, there are a number of cases of individuals with smaller parietal lesions who have more specific problems. For example, some individuals lose the ability to direct their arm toward visual targets but can nevertheless still make accurate saccadic eye movements toward the same targets. Conversely, there are instances of individuals who can reach out and touch visual targets that they cannot direct their gaze towards.

There are also cases of patients who can reach toward an object, but not shape their fingers into the appropriate grasp to pick it up—and vice versa. Being impaired at reaching accurately while still able to use visual information to form an appropriate hand grasp may be termed pure "optic ataxia." We introduced our patient Morris Harvey in Chapter 3—he has a unilateral optic ataxia from damage to his left (but not his right) hemisphere. Morris provides a good example of a pure optic ataxia—although it didn't seem that way at first. Morris doesn't tailor his grip size when reaching out for distant objects of different sizes—instead he adopts a wide-open hand posture whatever the size of the object. But Cristiana Cavina-Pratesi, working in our lab, has shown that when the object is literally close at hand and he doesn't need to move his arm to it, Morris's grip-scaling is perfectly normal. It seems that it is only when he is apt to miss the target due to his inaccurate reaching that he doesn't scale his grip. In other words, this is not really a failure to scale, it is a compensatory strategy; whatever the object, he plays it safe and opens his hand wide when the object is far away. His apparent failure to tailor his grasp is secondary to his misreaching, not a primary disorder of grasping per se.

We now know that the dorsal stream in humans is located mostly within and around the intraparietal sulcus, which runs roughly horizontally along the upper region of the parietal lobe (see Figure 5.9). Functional brain imaging has shown that there are separate areas in this posterior parietal region that are specialized for reaching, saccadic eye movements, and grasping, lined up in that order from the back part of this region to the front end (just like they are in the monkey brain, see Chapter 4, Figure 4.10). For example, a healthy person lying in the MRI scanner can be shown lights in different locations on a computer screen, and asked on each occasion either to turn his gaze to the light, or to reach out to it. When the person has to make reaching movements, the first of these areas (the superior parieto-occipital

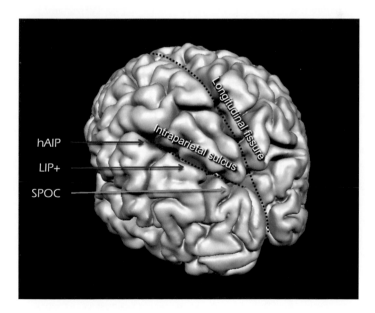

Figure 5.9 The locations of the human homologs of areas in the monkey brain that are specialized for different kinds of visually guided movements. These fMRI-defined regions include the superior parieto-occipital cortex (SPOC), which is thought to correspond to V6A, LIP+ (corresponding to monkey LIP), and hAIP (corresponding to AIP). These human areas have been shown to be activated during visually guided reaching, saccadic eye movements, and grasping, respectively.

cortex, or SPOC, the human version of area V6A in the monkey) is activated. In contrast, when the person has to look at the very same target rather than reach to it, the next area in line (the human lateral intraparietal area, or LIP+) is activated instead. If the person moved both his eyes *and* his hand when pointing to the target (the natural way of doing it) then both areas would be activated.

To determine which area becomes specifically activated when a visible target object is grasped, it is necessary to subtract out the areas of activation that might result from the eye movements and reaching that usually occur at the same time (see Box 5.1 for an example of this subtraction method). This is done by getting the person to keep their eyes steady at all times, and then by subtracting the brain's activation pattern for reaching toward objects from the pattern obtained during reaching for *and grasping* the same objects. When this is done, only the frontmost of the three areas (the human anterior intraparietal area, hAIP) shows a net increase in activity. It is worth noting again that all of these three areas—for reaches, quick eye movements (saccades), and grasps—have very close homologs that were identified in and around the monkey's intraparietal sulcus (see Chapter 4) long before they were discovered in humans.

The separate contributions of two of these areas, hAIP and SPOC, was nicely confirmed in some recent experiments by Cristiana Cavina-Pratesi and Jody Culham at the University of Western Ontario, Canada. As we mentioned earlier when discussing work with the optic ataxia patient Morris Harvey, a neat way to tease apart the two basic components of a reaching-and-grasping movement in human subjects is to test for grasping when no reach is required—that is, when the object is so close to the hand that only one's hand and wrist need to move to grab the object. Cavina-Pratesi and Culham used this trick to examine the activity in the separate brain areas concerned with controlling the reach and grasp components in the human dorsal stream. By comparing close versus far actions, they were able to confirm the specificity of the SPOC area for the reach component and the hAIP area for the grasp component: SPOC was activated only for far actions, where a reach was required, whereas hAIP was activated by grasps made to objects both close-to-hand and at a distance (see Figure 5.10). This clear dissociation between hAIP and SPOC provides an immediate explanation for why patients with optic ataxia may or may not have an associated primary deficit in grip formation—it all depends on the pattern and extent of dorsal-stream damage in each individual patient.

TMS (see Box 5.3) also has shed light on the functions of different areas in the human dorsal stream. In 1999, Michel Desmurget, a neuroscientist working in Lyon, France, showed that applying TMS to a particular region in the posterior parietal cortex of healthy volunteers disrupted their ability to adjust their reaching movements online to deal with a sudden shift in the position of the target. This result nicely confirms the demonstration by Yves Rossetti's group that optic ataxia patients

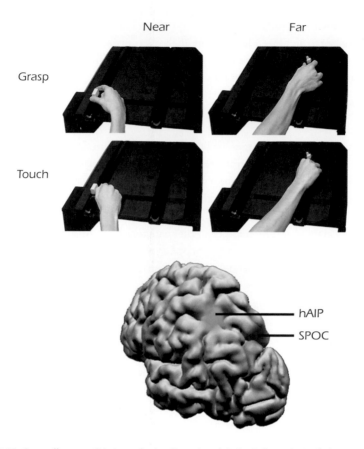

Figure 5.10 Our colleagues Cristiana Cavina-Pratesi and Jody Culham devised the arrangement shown at the top to separate out the "reach" and "grasp" components of a person's action when reaching to pick up an object. Both the starting point and the object location were varied, so that volunteers would have to make either a "far" or a "near" action on different occasions. In the "near" grasping task, the volunteer did not have to move the arm at all—the hand was already where it needed to be to grasp the object. Area SPOC was activated only during "far" reaches, whereas area hAIP was activated during both near and far reaches. Reprinted from Cavina-Pratesi, C., Monaco, S., Fattori, P., Galletti, C., McAdam, T.D., Quinlan, D.J., Goodale, M.A., and Culham, J.C., Functional magnetic resonance imaging reveals the neural substrates of arm transport and grip formation in reach-to-grasp actions in humans. *Journal of Neuroscience, 30*, 10306–10323, Figure 1. © 2010, Society for Neuroscience, with permission.

who have lesions in this same region of the posterior parietal cortex are unable to make these kinds of rapid automatic corrections to their movements (see Chapter 3). In more recent studies, Scott Grafton, then at Dartmouth College, New Hampshire, USA, has used TMS to confirm the role of area hAIP in grasping. The application of TMS to this area produces a disruption of grip scaling while a healthy person is reaching to grasp an object. In addition, there is a suggestion that applying TMS to the left hAIP interferes with visually guided grasping in the right hand rather than the left (and vice versa).

Summary

We have seen in this chapter that the broad divisions within the visual brain, the ventral and dorsal streams, are themselves subdivided into smaller modules, each with a specific job to do—either providing a specific kind of visual perception, in the case of the ventral stream, or guiding a specific kind of movement, in the case of the dorsal stream. The modularity in the ventral stream presumably reflects the fact that making distinctions within different perceptual categories requires that different kinds of information be extracted from the incoming visual signals. The modularity in the dorsal stream, however, is dictated by the need to convert visual information into different kinds of actions.

The findings of the brain imaging studies reviewed in this chapter mesh nicely with the results of behavioral and psychological studies of neurological patients. The imaging studies, however, as accurate as they are in pinpointing areas that appear to be related to particular visual functions, cannot by themselves tell us anything about the causal role of those areas in visual perception and visuomotor performance. Research with brain-damaged patients can do this—but the conclusions are almost always limited by the fact that brain damage does not respect functional boundaries. In Chapter 6, we shall address this issue more directly by introducing recent brain imaging work carried out with Dee and other brain-damaged patients as well healthy volunteers. These kinds of studies, combining the lesion method with brain imaging, provide an opportunity to look at the brain activity in patients while they are being tested not only on visual tasks where they do well but also on tasks in which they are clearly impaired. Moreover, as we shall see, the application of structural brain imaging to the plotting of lesions across patients with the same kinds of behavioral deficits has made it possible to narrow down the critical areas responsible for the observed impairments.

Further Reading

Martha Farah's book on visual agnosia provides an excellent overview of the higher-level deficits in perception that can follow damage to the ventral stream and other brain areas:

Farah, M.J. (2004). *Visual Agnosia* (2nd edition). Cambridge, MA: MIT Press/ Bradford Books.

This edited collection of case studies further illustrates the broad range of selective deficits in perception that have been described in the neurological and neuropsychological literature:

Humphreys, G.W. (2001). *Case Studies in the Neuropsychology of Vision*. London: Psychology Press.

For an engaging and first-hand clinical account of the variety of visual disorders that can arise from different kinds of brain damage, the reader is encouraged to read the following two books by Oliver Sacks:

Sacks, O. (1985). *The Man who Mistook his Wife for a Hat*. New York, NY: Summit Books.

Sacks, O. (1995). *An Anthropologist on Mars*. New York, NY: Alfred A. Knopf.

The following paper by Morris Moscovitch and colleagues describes Charles K., a man with visual object agnosia but intact imagery and face recognition:

Moscovitch, M., Winocur, G., and Behrmann, M. (1997). What is special about face recognition? Nineteen experiments on a person with visual object agnosia and dyslexia but normal face recognition. *Journal of Cognitive Neuroscience, 9,* 555–604.

For a discussion of face perception in general, see:

Bruce, V. and Young, A.W. (1998). *In the Eye of the Beholder: The science of face perception*. New York, NY: Oxford University Press.

The following article summarizes the current state of play in understanding the brain areas concerned with face perception:

Atkinson, A.P. and Adolphs, R. (2011). The neuropsychology of face perception: beyond simple dissociations and functional selectivity. *Philosophical Transactions of the Royal Society of London B (Biological Sciences), 366,* 1726–1738.

The following papers provide reviews of the functional organization of the human dorsal and ventral streams as revealed by fMRI:

Culham, J.C. and Valyear, K.F. (2006). Human parietal cortex in action. *Current Opinion in Neurobiology, 16,* 205–212.

Goodale, M.A. (2011). Transforming vision into action. *Vision Research, 51,* 1567–1587.

Grill-Spector, K. (2003). The neural basis of object perception. *Current Opinion in Neurobiology, 13,* 159–166.

Malach, R., Levy, I., and Hasson, U. (2002). The topography of high-order human object areas. *Trends in Cognitive Sciences*, 6, 176–184.

For readers who would like to know more about how fMRI can be used to study a range of psychological phenomena, the following book provides an excellent overview:

Huettel, S.A., Song, A.W., and McCarthy, G. (2009). *Functional Magnetic Resonance Imaging* (2nd edition). Sunderland, MA: Sinauer Associates.

The reader can learn more about the use of TMS from consulting these articles—the first a classic review of the technique, and the other a summary of how its use converges with fMRI in the study of vision:

McKeefry, D.J., Gouws, A., Burton, M.P., and Morland, A.B. (2009). The noninvasive dissection of the human visual cortex: using FMRI and TMS to study the organization of the visual brain. *Neuroscientist*, 15, 489–506.

Walsh, V. and Cowey, A. (2000). Transcranial magnetic stimulation and cognitive neuroscience. *Nature Reviews Neuroscience*, 1, 73–79.

VI

The anatomy of conscious and unconscious vision

The development of neuroimaging and its ever-advancing sophistication has not only allowed us to make fascinating and important discoveries about the normal brain, it has also allowed us to throw new light on the brains of patients whose behavior has long intrigued investigators like ourselves. In this chapter we will review how structural and functional neuroimaging have contributed to our understanding of three kinds of visual impairment that are of central importance to this book—optic ataxia, visual form agnosia, and hemianopia.

Neuroimaging of optic ataxia and visual form agnosia

Characterizing the damage that causes the visuomotor difficulties encountered by patients like Ruth Vickers and Anne Thiérry is relatively easy—they all have clearly defined damage that can be seen on structural scans such as computed tomography or magnetic resonance imaging (MRI) to include the region in and around the intra-parietal sulcus (IPS) in the upper parts of the parietal lobe. Indeed it was from this fact—documented by Perenin and Vighetto during the 1980s—that it was first possible to infer that the human dorsal stream terminates in the region of the IPS. A subsequent collaboration between Perenin and Hans-Otto Karnath has narrowed the critical area down to what they called the "parieto-occipital junction" (POJ) at the back end of the IPS—an area that appears to correspond reasonably well with the area now called SPOC (see Chapter 5). They did this by plotting the overlap between damaged brain territories in a series of patients *with* optic ataxia, and subtracting from this the regions of overlap among a control series of patients *without* optic ataxia. Interestingly, Perenin and her collaborators have found using functional MRI (fMRI) that this same area is activated in healthy volunteers reaching toward targets in peripheral vision (that is, targets away from their line of sight). In contrast, when people reached toward targets in central vision, a separate region in the IPS anterior and lateral to SPOC was activated instead. These results would explain why some patients with optic ataxia have problems only with peripheral targets, while others with wider areas of damage, like Anne Thiérry, also make errors with central targets.

The story, however, is not so straightforward in the case of Dee and her brain damage. In the case of optic ataxia, numerous patients can be scanned who have relatively discrete damage, mostly caused by stroke (either a blockage in the blood supply to a particular brain region or a ruptured blood vessel). This has allowed "lesion overlap" analyses to be done. Dee's brain damage is much less clearly defined than this, since it resulted from carbon monoxide poisoning, a form of pathology that has widespread effects throughout the brain. Yet she certainly does not have uniform damage throughout her visual system. As we saw earlier in the book, structural MRI scans taken in hospital soon after her accident showed that a large part of her primary visual cortex, V1, was still intact, although there was damage in the lower part of her occipital and temporal lobes on both sides. More than a decade later, we obtained more detailed MRI information about the damage to Dee's brain in collaboration with Tom James and Jody Culham, using a powerful brain scanner at the Robarts Research Institute in London, Ontario. These studies allowed us to look for the first time at the actual workings of Dee's visual system, and not only at the structural damage it has suffered. We carried out a systematic series of brain scans, requiring Dee to spend time inside the magnet not just once but for several scanning sessions. It is not pleasant for anyone to have to keep completely still in the confined space of the bore of the magnet for periods of more than thirty minutes at a time. Not only is the inside of the magnet dark and oppressive, particularly for someone like Dee who is already a bit claustrophobic, but it is very noisy as well. Nevertheless, Dee persevered and overcame her reluctance with real fortitude, and we were able to obtain some excellent structural images of her brain as well as a whole series of functional images.

The structural scan revealed a particularly dense lesion on both sides of her brain in what we now know as area LO (see Chapter 5, Figure 5.8)—in the same general region that had been identified as abnormal in the MRI scans taken a decade earlier. To explore this we went on to carry out a fMRI study in which we contrasted the pattern of brain activation that occurred when first healthy volunteers, and then Dee herself, looked at pictures of real objects with the activation that occurred when they looked at scrambled versions of those same pictures. As we saw in Chapter 5, the differences between the brain activations generated by these two different sets of pictures should reveal the areas specific for processing object shape, that is, area LO. They should also reveal whether or not these net activations are normal in Dee's brain. Needless to say, we used line drawings because the only route to identifying them was through their shape and form, which is precisely where Dee has a problem.

As expected, the brains of our healthy volunteers showed a robust activation in area LO, which we could then compare against the damaged area we had already seen in Dee's brain. The two areas corresponded remarkably well (Figure 6.1). The correspondence became even more evident when the activation in a control subject's brain was mathematically superimposed onto a section through Dee's brain (Figure 6.2, right). This activity fell neatly within the areas of lost tissue on both sides of her brain, suggesting that area LO was essentially missing in her brain. In

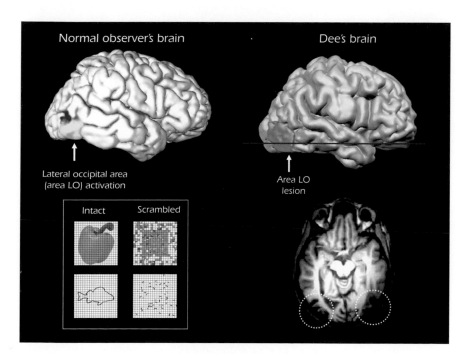

Figure 6.1 The left half of this figure shows the differential activation in area LO in a normal observer viewing intact versus scrambled images of objects. The top right-hand picture shows the location of Dee's lesion in the ventral stream. Remarkably, her lesion sits exactly where area LO is found in the normal brain. The section through her brain (shown below) at the level of the red line shows that similar lesions in the territory of area LO are present on both sides.

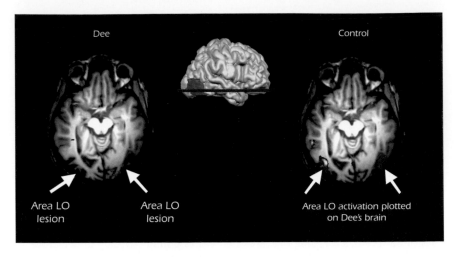

Figure 6.2 The horizontal section on the left (at the level of the red line) shows the fMRI activation in Dee's brain as she looks at line drawings (versus scrambled drawings). Note that there is no selective activation for the intact drawings either in area LO or in neighboring areas in her brain. In contrast, control observers show robust activations to the same drawings. The activation in one of these observer's brains, which has been mathematically morphed to fit onto Dee's brain, coincides well with her LO lesions. Reprinted from Thomas W. James, Jody Culham, G. Keith Humphrey, A. David Milner, and Melvyn A. Goodale, Ventral occipital lesions impair object recognition but not object-directed grasping: an fMRI study, *Brain*, 2003, *126*(11), 2463–2475, Figure 4, with permission from Oxford University Press.

a convincing confirmation of this, there was no differential activation *anywhere* in Dee's ventral stream when she looked at line drawings of objects. In other words, the patterns of activation in her ventral stream elicited by line drawings of objects were indistinguishable from those elicited by the scrambled versions (Figure 6.2, left). Just as we had inferred from our original testing many years earlier, her brain registers the presence of lines and edges at early levels of the visual system, but due to the damage in her ventral stream it cannot put these elements together to form perceived "wholes."

These striking findings permit a much more confident interpretation of Dee's visual form agnosia. In a nutshell, Dee lacks the crucial area that normally allows us to see that a drawing represents a particular whole object rather than a meaningless fragmented one. Without area LO, we lose our ability to see the structure or "gestalt" that distinguishes a particular whole from simply a set of component elements.

Although Dee is essentially shape-blind, she can nevertheless name many objects on the basis of their color and visual texture, when those surface properties are diagnostic of their identity. So our next step was to test Dee in the scanner with colored photographs of objects in which all the surface features of the object were present: color, visual texture, and reflective highlights. This time the pattern of activation that we observed was very different. The activation from the colored photographs (compared to scrambled versions of the same photographs) was not in area LO (which of course was badly damaged in Dee) but was located instead in neighboring regions of the ventral stream (see Figure 6.3, right). Similar regions were activated to some extent in our healthy volunteers, in their case along with a strong activation of area LO. It is worth noting that these wider activations were not just produced by color per se—after all, the scrambled pictures were colored too, and the activations from them had been subtracted in the patterns of activation we were looking at. Instead, what we are seeing is the activation of networks that actually participate in Dee's perception of *colored objects*. In confirmation of this idea, we found that

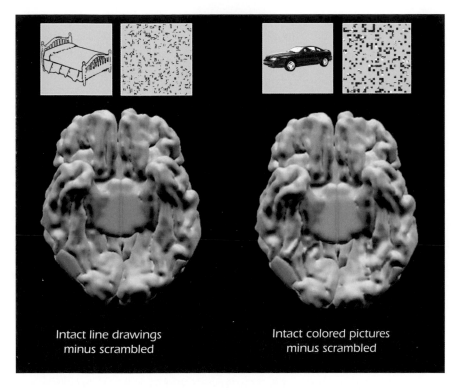

Intact line drawings
minus scrambled

Intact colored pictures
minus scrambled

Figure 6.3 Shown here are ventral views of Dee's brain. Although her brain shows no differential activation for black and white line drawings (left-hand picture), it does show robust activation for full color photographs of objects (right-hand picture). Of course, these activations arise in brain areas that are spared in Dee, in more medial and anterior parts of her ventral stream.

the extent of activation of these areas correlated strongly with her success in naming the objects—the stronger the activation on a given presentation, the better she did. Most probably the color and other surface features of the objects depicted in the intact pictures, to the extent to which they are diagnostic of what the objects are, allow her brain to extract the "stuff" or material properties (plastic, metal, wood, fur, etc.) of the objects, and go from there to a correct identification (see Chapter 5, Figure 5.6).

Research by our colleague Jennifer Steeves, now at York University in Canada, suggests that Dee can make good use of her spared color and texture perception, not only to identify objects on the basis of their surface properties but also to recognize scenes. Steeves found that Dee is remarkably good at categorizing colored photographs of scenes (forests vs. cityscapes vs. beaches etc.) and also showed robust activation in the parahippocampal place area (PPA) when presented with these same pictures in the fMRI magnet. Not surprisingly, Dee has great difficulty categorizing these same scenes when they are presented as black and white drawings—and the activity in her PPA is virtually absent when she views these same drawings. Normal individuals of course show robust activation in the PPA with either colored photographs or black and white drawings—and have no trouble categorizing them correctly.

The results of the studies with line drawings and colored photographs not only help us to understand what Dee has *lost* (her ability to see shape and form), but also to gain insights into what she has *retained*. Together, the research has allowed us to map out the areas in the ventral stream that are still functioning in Dee's brain and those that are not. The activations evoked by colored photographs (see Figure 6.3) strongly suggest that some of the specialized perceptual systems in her temporal lobes for recognizing objects must be still receiving and interpreting visual messages, even though they are not getting information about the *shape* of those objects. Although this at present remains a fascinating puzzle, we have got some important insights into what is going on from a series of studies carried out by Cristiana Cavina-Pratesi, who compared activations in Dee's brain with those in the achromatopsic patient Martin Smithson, whom we introduced in the last chapter.

Cavina-Pratesi showed that the spared areas in Dee's ventral stream showed responses to colors and textures but not to shape, whereas the areas that remain intact in Martin Smithson's brain showed responses to shape but not to color or texture. Importantly, the "shape areas" in Martin's brain corresponded with those in the healthy brain: namely, area LO (Figure 6.4). Likewise, the areas that were sensitive to color and texture in Dee's brain were in the same anatomical location as those seen in the healthy controls, but in this case, regions that were more medial and anterior to area LO (see Figure 6.5). These findings join an increasing number of

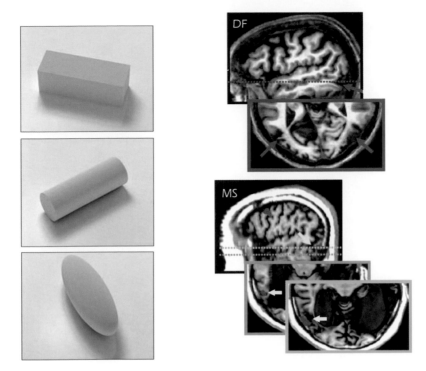

Figure 6.4 This figure and Figure 6.5 summarize the results of a study by Cristiana Cavina-Pratesi and her colleagues that examined the activity in Dee's brain (DF) and also in Martin Smithson's (MS), as each of them viewed images of objects that differed in either shape (this figure) or surface texture (Figure 6.5). On the right, one can see horizontal sections through the back of Dee and Martin's brains (in the planes indicated by the dotted lines in corresponding colors). These sections pass through the normal location of area LO, present in Martin (yellow arrows) but missing in Dee (indicated by the purple arrows). Not surprisingly, only Martin shows any indication of shape-related activity. Reprinted from C. Cavina-Pratesi, R.W. Kentridge, C.A. Heywood, and A.D. Milner, Separate processing of texture and form in the ventral stream: evidence from fMRI and visual agnosia, *Cerebral Cortex*, 2010, 20(2), 433–446, Figures 1 and 7, with permission from Oxford University Press.

studies showing that the processing of object form involves a quite separate network in the ventral stream from that processing the surface properties of objects. But they go further by providing evidence that these networks are *necessary* for the perception of those respective properties.

A simpler story emerged when we looked at brain activations in Dee's dorsal stream. Here we were examining not the parts of her visual brain that we assumed were damaged, but instead the parts that seemed to be working well. We used a piece of equipment devised by Jody Culham, known affectionately as the "grasparatus"

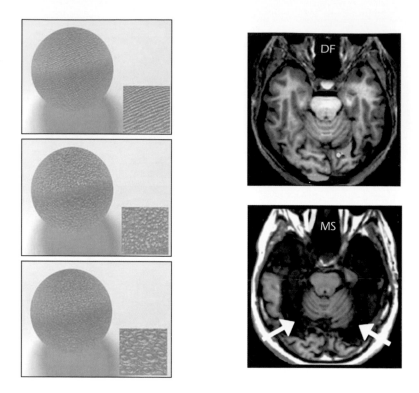

Figure 6.5 Here we see two horizontal sections through the ventral part of the occipital lobe in Dee and Martin's brains. At this level of the brain, we would normally expect to see activation that is selective for surface texture. But only Dee's brain shows any evidence of such activation. In Martin's brain, we see no activation as the critical region for surface texture is clearly missing (indicated by white arrows). Reprinted from C. Cavina-Pratesi, R.W. Kentridge, C.A. Heywood, and A.D. Milner, Separate processing of texture and form in the ventral stream: evidence from fMRI and visual agnosia, *Cerebral Cortex*, 2010, 20(2), 433–446, Figure 8, with by permission from Oxford University Press.

(see Figure 6.6), to identify which areas in Dee's brain became active when she reached out and grasped small blocks presented to her in the scanner—and how these areas corresponded to those that were active in the brains of healthy volunteers doing the same task (see Figure 6.7).

The results nicely confirmed our earlier speculations—that is, we found that, just as in our normal volunteers, Dee's brain showed activation in area hAIP, at the anterior end of the IPS (Figure 6.8). As we noted in earlier chapters, this part of the human dorsal stream appears to correspond closely to the similarly-located area AIP in the monkey, which is known to be intimately associated with the visual control of grasping. Thus, in retrospect, we can understand clearly why Dee retains the

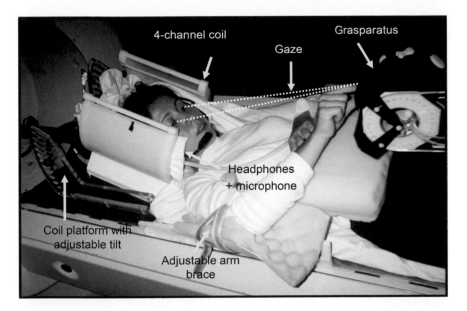

Figure 6.6 The "grasparatus" used in Jody Culham's laboratory. The person lies with the head tilted, looking directly at an eight-sided drum that can be rotated pneumatically. A number of different three-dimensional objects can be presented at any one time on each face of the drum. The person can easily reach out and touch or grasp whichever object is illuminated. (Note that the experiment would normally be run in the dark with only the goal object visible.) The grasparatus contains no ferromagnetic (e.g. steel) components, to avoid problems with the strong magnetic field within the scanner.

ability to grasp objects of different sizes and shapes: the dorsal-stream area that is responsible for the visual guidance of grasping evidently continues to work normally in her brain.

Optic ataxic patients are not the mirror image of Dee

We know from structural MRI studies that patients with optic ataxia have damage to the critical region for visually guided reaching, namely SPOC. But some of these patients, those that also have a real deficit in grasping, presumably also have further damage in the dorsal stream, including hAIP. It is only patients with such damage to hAIP that provide an informative double dissociation with Dee: whereas patients with hAIP damage can perceive the shape of objects but cannot grasp them properly, Dee can grasp them but cannot perceive their shape. Optic ataxia itself, which is defined as a reaching deficit to objects in visual space, is not mirrored exactly in Dee's clinical picture. Her visual form agnosia is not primarily a disorder of visual

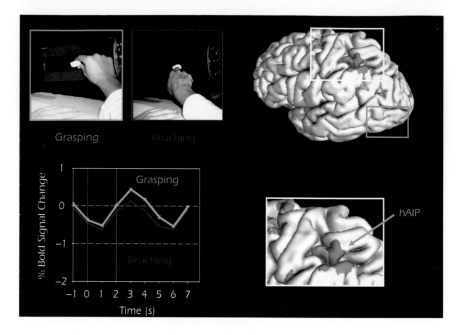

Figure 6.7 The graph at the bottom left side shows the time course of activations in hAIP when a healthy volunteer reached out and grasped the object (green) versus when she reached out and touched the object without forming a grasp (red). The location of hAIP is mapped onto the left hemisphere of the brain (and inset) on the right side of the figure. (The other grasp-specific activations shown on the brain are in motor and somatosensory cortex.) Note that in area LO (surrounded by the blue rectangle) there is no differential activation for grasping. Adapted from Thomas W. James, Jody Culham, G. Keith Humphrey, A. David Milner, Melvyn A. Goodale, Ventral occipital lesions impair object recognition but not object-directed grasping: an fMRI study, *Brain*, 2003, *126*(11), pp. 2463–2475, Figure 7, by permission of Oxford University Press.

space perception; it's a disorder of form or shape perception. In short, it is important to realize that damage to the dorsal stream can result in many different visuomotor deficits just as ventral-stream damage can result in many different perceptual deficits. The most compelling double dissociations between damage to the dorsal and ventral stream comes from patients who, when faced with the same visual array, can use the information to perform task A but not task B, or vice versa.

Classic optic ataxia, as defined in neurology, is a disorder of reaching. Since we now know that different areas in the dorsal stream are responsible for different kinds of visuomotor behavior, perhaps we need a new nomenclature that reflects the fact that patients with damage to the dorsal stream can have quite different clusters of impairments. Some will have difficulty in reaching but not grasping, for example, and others will have difficulty in the control of eye movements but not in reaching or grasping. And of course some, like Anne Thiérry with classic Bálint's syndrome, will have deficits in the visual guidance of all these movements.

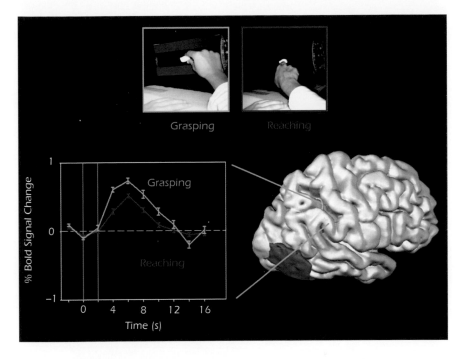

Figure 6.8 Activations in Dee's brain during reaching and grasping. Right: The activation corresponding to grasping vs. reaching is shown in green in in Dee's brain, in a location that is in the same location as hAIP in the intact brain. Left: The averaged time-course of activations for grasping and reaching trials in hAIP. Clearly, hAIP is functioning normally in spite of Dee's brain damage. (The large lesion in Dee's area LO is indicated in dark gray.) Adapted from Thomas W. James, Jody Culham, G. Keith Humphrey, A. David Milner, Melvyn A. Goodale, Ventral occipital lesions impair object recognition but not object-directed grasping: an fMRI study, *Brain*, 2003, *126*(11), pp. 2463–2475, Figure 7, by permission of Oxford University Press.

"Blindsight"

Dee has given us some particularly striking and powerful examples of preserved visuomotor control despite profound perceptual disability. Historically speaking, she was the source of inspiration for much of the theory and research that we are summarizing in this book. But she is by no means the first brain-damaged patient in the literature to show "action without perception." Some years before we encountered Dee, investigators had discovered a similar and equally striking contrast between visual experience and visuomotor control—but in patients with a rather different kind of brain damage.

As can be seen in Figure 6.9, the left hemisphere sees only the right half of the visual field, and the right hemisphere only the left. So when a patient sustains damage

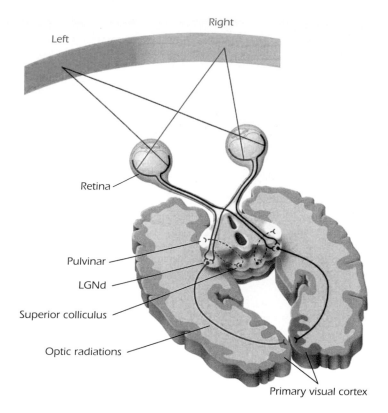

Figure 6.9 As this diagram shows, the left side of each retina, and eventually the left side of the brain too, sees the right side of the visual field. This route is coded as green in the diagram. The same holds for right side of each retina and the brain (coded as red). This means, for example, that damage to V1 on the left causes subjective blindness in the right half of the visual field, in both eyes.

to either the primary visual cortex (V1), or the axons entering V1 from the lateral geniculate nucleus in the thalamus on one side of the brain, they are left with an apparently complete blindness in the visual field on the opposite side, in both eyes. The usual way to diagnose this half-blindness (hemianopia) in the clinic is to use a large circular screen or "perimeter," on which spots of light are flashed at different points while the patient holds his or her gaze steady on a central point on the screen. Hemianopic patients report seeing none of the spots of light that are flashed on the side of the screen opposite their brain damage.

We saw in Chapter 4 that the primate perceptual system resides in the ventral stream of visual processing, which passes from V1 down into the inferior regions of the occipital and temporal lobes. Part of the evidence for this was the research of Charles Gross and his colleagues, who recorded the electrical activity of neurons in the inferior temporal lobe in monkeys. As we mentioned in Chapter 4, they found that neurons in this region responded selectively to a whole range of different complex visual patterns and objects. Presumably the high-level properties of these neurons are the result of converging inputs from neurons at lower levels of the visual system that respond to the different visual features, such as shape, color, and visual texture, which define the objects. Gross and his colleagues went on to show unequivocally that the critical visual input to this form analysis system comes from V1. They did this by removing V1 in some monkeys, and showing that the cells in the inferior temporal cortex now remained "silent" whatever patterns were shown to the eye. So if the human ventral stream is like that of the monkey's, it will "see" nothing when V1 is damaged. This would explain why patients with this kind of damage have no visual experience in the affected part of the visual field.

However, Larry Weiskrantz, a neuropsychologist at the University of Oxford, UK, pointed out a strange paradox. Monkeys with damage to V1, who should just be as blind as these hemianopic humans, *could* detect visual input presented to their "blind" field. How could this be? One view at the time was that area V1 must have become more important for vision in humans than it was in our primate ancestors. According to the argument, this heavy reliance on V1 did not emerge in the evolution of present-day monkeys. Weiskrantz was reluctant to accept this idea since everything else that was known about the monkey's visual system showed that it was remarkably similar to that of the human. He realized that there was a simpler way to resolve this paradox—one that respected the evolutionary kinship between monkey and human. As Weiskrantz pointed out, monkeys were never asked to *report* on what they saw; instead, they were simply trained to choose between two different visual displays or to reach out and grasp a piece of food. In contrast, the human patients were really being asked to comment on their *experience*: Did they *see* something out there in the world? All the monkeys cared about was getting their food reward for responding correctly. Weiskrantz suggested that the monkeys with lesions of V1 might be achieving this without having any conscious visual experience at all. As far as they were concerned, they were just guessing—and when they guessed correctly they got rewarded. Perhaps humans, he suggested, could be tested in exactly the same way. In other words, if the patients were not asked "Did you see the light?" but instead were asked to reach toward it, perhaps they too would show the same spared visual sensitivity as the monkey with V1 lesions.

When patients with V1 lesions began to be tested in this way, a whole panoply of spared visual abilities was uncovered. Patients could point accurately or move their gaze toward targets that they insisted they couldn't see. For example, Rob Whitwell and Chris Striemer in our laboratory have been testing a patient, Susan James, who had a stroke on the left side of her brain. An MRI scan showed that she had a large area of damage in her left V1 (see Figure 6.10). The lesion has left her with a dense hemianopia in her right visual field. Yet despite her apparent blindness, Susan was able to point well above chance to small targets presented briefly in the "blind" right visual field (see Figure 6.11). In other words she could point to things that she insisted she couldn't see.

During the 1990s, Marie-Thérèse Perenin and Yves Rossetti found that some patients could even scale their grip and correctly rotate their wrist when reaching out to grasp objects placed in their "blind" field. We were interested to investigate whether Susan James could do this too. So Rob and Chris first presented her with small rectangular objects of different widths in her blind field and asked her to estimate their width by opening her finger and thumb a matching amount. Like Dee

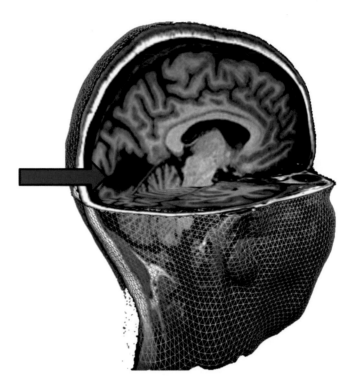

Figure 6.10 Structural MRI scan of Susan James's brain, rendered in three dimensions. Susan's brain damage (arrow) is largely restricted to the early visual areas, including all of area V1. Reprinted from *Vision Research*, *51*(8), Robert L. Whitwell, Christopher L. Striemer, David A. Nicolle, and Melvyn A. Goodale, Grasping the non-conscious: preserved grip scaling to unseen objects for immediate but not delayed grasping following a unilateral lesion to primary visual cortex, pp. 908–924, Figure 1. © (2011), with permission from Elsevier.

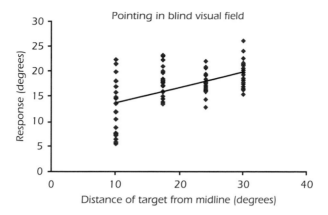

Figure 6.11 This graph shows where Susan's finger ended up when she was asked to point to targets briefly flashed in her blind field. Even though Susan was far from perfect, there was a clear correlation between her responses and the target locations: the further out the target was in her blind field, the further out she pointed. Reprinted from *Vision Research*, 51(8), Robert L. Whitwell, Christopher L. Striemer, David A. Nicolle, and Melvyn A. Goodale, Grasping the non-conscious: preserved grip scaling to unseen objects for immediate but not delayed grasping following a unilateral lesion to primary visual cortex, pp. 908–924, Figure 2. © (2011), with permission from Elsevier.

(see Chapter 2) she failed completely. But again like Dee, when Susan reached out to grasp the objects (which she again adamantly denied seeing), her finger–thumb aperture opened in flight in a way that was clearly affected by the width of the object. Admittedly, her grip scaling was not nearly as good as that shown by Dee. Nevertheless, here we have a case of an individual without V1 who can still use visual information to control skilled actions such as grasping, albeit not as well as normal people.

In another recent study in our laboratory of a patient with V1 damage, Chris Striemer and Craig Chapman used the obstacle avoidance task described in Chapter 3, and found that efficient visuomotor processing of an "unseen" object could occur in this context as well. In other words, the patient took avoidance action in relation to a potential obstacle in his blind field just as if he could see it perfectly well, even though he consistently denied seeing anything at all in that visual field.

In all these cases, then, asking patients with V1 damage to perform an action, rather than report their experience, revealed unsuspected but impressive visual capacities regarding objects that they adamantly denied seeing. Weiskrantz coined the whimsical term "blindsight" to refer to all of these various preserved visual capacities in the "blind" field.

So what is going on here? How is it that blindsight patients, and indeed monkeys with V1 lesions, can do these things? After all, the brain damage they have suffered would appear to have closed the front door between the eye and the two cortical visual streams. One clue is that for the most part the preserved abilities are visuomotor in nature. This raises the possibility that more ancient sensorimotor structures, like the superior colliculus, could be involved. The pathway from the eye to these brainstem structures would not be disrupted by the brain damage suffered by "blindsight" patients, so visual input from the eyes could still get through to them (see Chapters 3 and 4). This would certainly explain how the patients can look toward things they say they cannot see, because the colliculus both receives visual signals directly from the eye and translates those signals directly into eye movements without any help from the cortex.

But this by itself would not account for the fact that blindsight patients can point to or even grasp objects presented in their "blind" field. These are activities that depend, as we saw earlier, on cortical systems in the dorsal stream. Without a working V1, how could visual information reach these dorsal stream systems? The answer seems to be that although the ventral stream depends entirely on V1 for its visual inputs, the dorsal stream does not. Back in the 1980s, the French neuroscientist Jean Bullier showed that neurons within the dorsal stream (quite unlike those in the ventral stream) still respond to visual inputs even when V1 is inactivated by cooling. The most likely route for this information to reach the dorsal stream is again via the superior colliculus, which in addition to its direct role in eye movement control is known to be a way-station along a major visual route from the eyes to the cerebral cortex. This "back-door" route entirely bypasses V1 and so would remain intact in blindsight patients (Figure 6.12).

Dee Fletcher's residual vision is ultimately not that different from blindsight. She has the advantage of retaining a largely intact area V1, giving her a much more efficient visual route to dorsal stream areas than the blindsight patient, who has to rely on the more primitive midbrain route alone. Dee is also less severely disabled than the blindsight patient in that only part of her visual experience has been lost—her perception of shape and form. But despite all this, she does resemble the blindsight patient in one important way: that she can perform many motor tasks under visual control while having no perceptual experience of the visual features controlling her behavior. And in both cases it is most likely that the brain machinery ultimately responsible for this preserved behavior is located in the dorsal stream.

Summary

In Chapters 4 and 5, we have seen that brain imaging offers a powerful tool for illuminating the functional anatomy of the visual system. All of this work together with the studies on brain-damaged patients and monkeys tells the same story: that

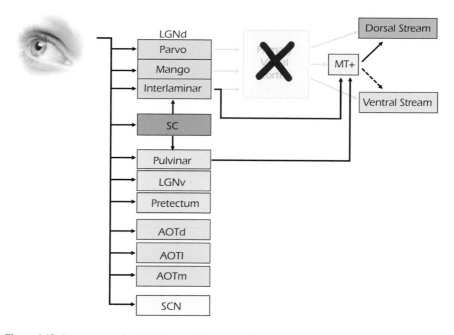

Figure 6.12 As we saw earlier (in Chapter 4, Box 4.1), the eye sends information to many different structures in the brain. Although primary visual cortex (V1) serves as the major conduit for input to the ventral and dorsal streams, after lesions of V1, information can still reach the cortex, particularly the dorsal stream, via other routes. These alternative routes can readily account for a good number of the spared abilities seen in blindsight.

the ventral and dorsal streams play very different, and complementary, roles in our visual life. But why is it this way? In Chapter 7, we will examine how the different demands of visual perception and the visual guidance of action have led to the evolution of two distinct visual streams in the primate brain.

Further Reading

This article describes our initial discoveries using fMRI of Dee's intact and impaired visual areas:

James, T.W., Culham, J., Humphrey, G.K., Milner, A.D., and Goodale, M.A. (2003). Ventral occipital lesions impair object recognition but not object-directed grasping: a fMRI study. *Brain*, *126*, 2463–2475.

This later fMRI and behavioral study explores Dee's ability to recognize scenes:

Steeves, J.K., Humphrey, G.K., Culham, J.C., Menon, R.S., Milner, A.D., and Goodale, M.A. (2004). Behavioral and neuroimaging evidence for a contribution of color and texture information to scene classification in a patient with visual form agnosia. *Journal of Cognitive Neuroscience, 16,* 955–965.

This paper describes the experiments demonstrating a double dissociation between Dee and Martin's abilities to perceive object shape and object texture:

Cavina-Pratesi, C., Kentridge, R.W., Heywood, C.A., and Milner A.D. (2010). Separate processing of texture and form in the ventral stream: evidence from fMRI and visual agnosia. *Cerebral Cortex, 20,* 433–446.

These two books by Larry Weiskrantz offer an authoritative account of blindsight and related disorders by a pioneer in the field:

Weiskrantz, L. (1990). *Blindsight: A case study and implications.* Oxford: Oxford University Press.

Weiskrantz, L. (1997). *Consciousness Lost and Found: A neuropsychological exploration.* Oxford: Oxford University Press.

The following two papers describe experiments with blindsight patients who can grasp and avoid objects that they cannot see:

Striemer, C.L., Chapman, C.S., and Goodale, M.A. (2009). "Real-time" obstacle avoidance in the absence of primary visual cortex. *Proceedings of the National Academy of Science of the United States of America, 106,* 15996–16001.

Whitwell, R.L., Striemer, C.L., Nicolle, D.A., and Goodale, M.A. (2011). Grasping the non-conscious: preserved grip scaling to unseen objects for immediate but not delayed grasping following a unilateral lesion to primary visual cortex. *Vision Research, 51,* 908–924.

VII

Why do we need two systems?

The evidence is clear that we humans have two visual systems in the cerebral cortex: one for perception and one for the visual control of action. We suggested in Chapter 4 that this division of labor must have emerged in our primate ancestors because of the different processing demands imposed by these two functions of vision. But what are these different demands of perception and action, and how are they reflected in the way the two streams deal with the visual input? What does perception need to know that the visual control of action does not—and vice versa?

First let us revisit for a moment what natural selection has "designed" the two systems to do. Visual perception is there to let us make sense of the outside world and to create representations of it in a form that can be filed away for future reference. In contrast, the control of a motor act—from picking up a morsel of food to throwing a spear at a fleeing antelope—requires accurate information about the actual size, location, and motion of the target object. This information has to be coded in the absolute metrics of the real world. In other words, it has to be coded in terms of the actual distance and size of the objects. In addition the information has to be available at the very instant the action has to be made.

These two broad objectives, as we shall argue in this chapter, impose such conflicting requirements on the brain that to deal with them within a single unitary visual system would present a computational nightmare.

A TV-watching module in the brain?

Perception puts objects in their context. We perceive the size, location, and motion of an object almost entirely in relation to other objects and surfaces in the scene. In other words, the metrics of perception are relative, not absolute—a fact that explains why we have no difficulty watching television, a medium in which there are no absolute metrics at all (Figure 7.1). Actually, the fact that we can follow what is happening on television is quite remarkable. All that we really see, after all, is patterns of light, shade, and color that are constantly shifting and changing over a small two-dimensional surface in front of us. Yet we have no trouble segregating these patterns into meaningful objects and making sense of the complex events the images represent.

The only metrical information that is available on TV is based on the relations between objects that are depicted on the screen, and our previous knowledge of their real geometry. Sometimes, for example, a face might fill the entire screen; on other occasions, it might be one of a sea of faces in a crowd. Yet in both cases we know that it is a face and we also know that it is closer in one case than the other. Worse still, there are unpredictable changes in the point of view. Here we are at the mercy of the camera operator, the editor, and the producer of the program—and yet, even with the fast jump-cuts and scene transitions that typify music videos and advertising, we have little trouble figuring out what is going on. The size, shape, and distance of objects can be inferred only from our knowledge of real-world geometry, from the relations among different objects in the scene, and from assumptions about continuity from one scene to the next. Despite all this, even young children have an immediate and natural understanding of what is unfolding on a TV screen.

Understanding television is not, of course, what our visual system evolved to do. We do not have a special "TV-watching module" in our brains. And yet television tells us something important about perception. Television simply would not have developed as a major medium for communication if our visual brain were not somehow receptive to the way in which it represents the world. There is little doubt that the brain mechanisms that allow us to watch and understand TV are the very same mechanisms that allow us to perceive and understand the real world. In real life too, the brain uses stored knowledge of everyday objects, such as their size, to make inferences about the sizes of other objects and about their distance from us and from each other. In order to extract the meaning and significance of the scene before us, we only need the relative size, position, and speed of the objects with respect to one another. We do not need to know the absolute metrics of every object in the scene in order to make sense of the visual world.

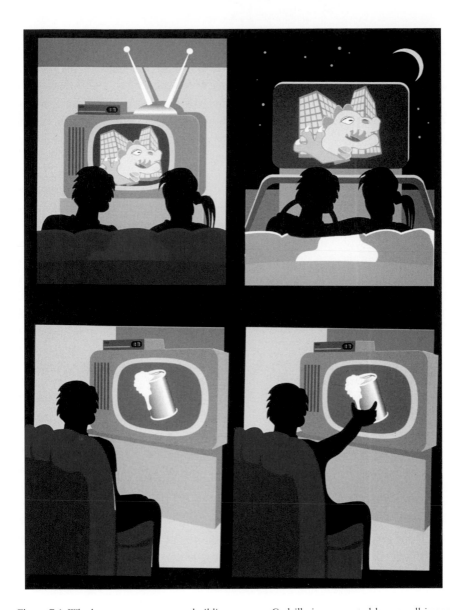

Figure 7.1 Whether or not a person, a building, or even Godzilla is represented by a small image on a TV screen or by a large image on a movie screen, is irrelevant to our understanding of what is going on. In fact, sometimes a person might fill the whole screen and sometimes be only a tiny figure running away from Godzilla. What matters to our perception is the *relative* size of people and things on the screen. But while we have no difficulty perceiving what is happening on the screen, we cannot reach out and grasp the things that are represented there. This is because the images do not reflect the real size and position of objects in the world. Watching television convincingly mimics our *experience* of the world. What it cannot mimic is the visual information that we need to act on the world.

In contrast, this kind of relative information is of little help in the control of action. To pick up a coffee cup, it is not enough to know that it is further away than the bowl of cornflakes and closer than the jar of marmalade; and knowing that the whole scene represents a breakfast table doesn't help much either. The brain systems that program and control our grasping movements must have access to accurate metrical information about the location of the cup and its real size. Furthermore, information about the cup's location and real distance must be computed in "egocentric" frames of reference—in other words, in relation to the observer rather than in relation to other objects.

Television can provide us with all kinds of useful general knowledge about the world around us, but it would be a hopeless medium for *acting* on things in the world. We might recognize a can of beer on a commercial but we could never pick it up—not just because it isn't real but because we see the beer can from the changing points of view of the camera operator and not from our own (see Figure 7.1). It is true that video images can be used successfully in a number of applications where humans are controlling robots or other instruments and a direct view of the workspace is not available. In these cases, however, the point of view and the magnification of the image are kept relatively constant. Imagine the disaster that would occur if a surgeon had to carry out a video-assisted operation in which the camera was moved around at the same speed and unpredictability as in a music video!

These arguments about the different requirements of perception and visually guided action lead to two important conclusions. First, since the computations leading to action must be metrically accurate (and highly reliable), they must depend on visual mechanisms that at some stage are quite separate from those mediating our perception of the world. Second, because different kinds of actions (e.g. manual grasping movements versus saccadic eye movements) require that the computations be performed within different egocentric frames of reference, there are likely to be several different visual mechanisms for the control of action, each specialized for the control of a different effector system (eyes, arm, leg, hand, fingers). As we have seen in the preceding chapters, nature seems to concur; that is, natural selection has created in primates a brain that embodies these design principles. To put it another way, the different computational demands of perception and action have presumably been a major driving force in the evolution of the visual brain (Box 7.1).

> **BOX 7.1** METRICS AND ACTING IN THE REAL WORLD
>
> We humans are active creatures. We are constantly interacting with objects in the world, from picking up our morning cup of coffee to hitting a golf ball with a well-practiced stroke. The question arises as to how the brain computes the locations of these objects. One possibility is

(Continued)

that it computes them on the spot using explicit metrics, i.e. in terms of distance and direction. Another equally plausible possibility is that the brain doesn't use an explicit metrical framework at all, but instead learns to make movements to targets by trial and error, and then retrieves the successful movements later when confronted with a target in the same location on a future occasion.

Much of the learning would take place while we are infants and children, but as we take up new activities, such as golf or soccer, then we have to refine these learned action routines. According to this view, it's not that the visuomotor systems in the brain code the actual distance and direction of the target for action on the spot, as much as calling up the required coordinates for that particular action from a set of stored motor coordinates that have been acquired through a lifetime. Of course, it is also possible that the brain uses both sorts of computations depending on the effector that is being used and the nature of the movement that is being made. Eye movements, for example, may use a very different coordinate system from that used by the reaching hand. Similarly, a well-practiced movement made toward a visible target may be more likely to make use of a stored motor routine than an unfamiliar movement made toward the same target. Moreover, actions such as throwing a dart, where the target is often several meters away from the body, may also depend more on recalling practiced movements than picking up an object in near space. What is certain is that however they are computed, to be successful, all these movements have to accurately reflect the real metrics of the world.

REFERENCE

Thaler L. and Goodale, M.A. (2010). Beyond distance and direction: the brain represents target locations non-metrically. *Journal of Vision, 10*(3), 3.

Time and the observer

Humans, like most other animals, rarely stay still for more than a few seconds at a time, except perhaps when they are sleeping. Indeed even when seated at our desk, we move our eyes around, swivel in our chair, and lean back and stretch occasionally. In other words, we rarely stay in a static relationship with objects that we may need to interact with. Yet we have no difficulty in reaching out and answering the phone, picking up our coffee cup, or shaking a colleague's hand when he or she comes into the room. We do all of these things, even though the patterns falling on the retinas of our eyes are constantly changing. Of course we "know," at one level, where the coffee cup is—it's on our desk, to the right of the telephone. But if we want to pick up the cup, our brain needs to compute exactly where the cup is with respect to our hand. Moreover, the brain has to come up with that information just as we are about to move. Relying on a computation made even two seconds earlier would be useless, except in the unlikely event that we (including our eyes) have remained completely immobile for that length of time. In other words the only way we can successfully and reliably guide a movement toward a goal object at a particular moment is by having continually updated visual information available to us. This means that the brain has to compute the precise parameters needed to specify an action immediately before the movements are to be initiated. By the same token it would make little sense to store this information for more than a fraction of a second, whether or not the action is actually performed. Not only would its value be strictly time-limited, it would be positively disadvantageous to keep the information hanging around in the system.

Of course it cannot be denied that we are well able to make reaching and grasping movements using "old" visual information, even after an object has been taken away—for example, we can pretend to grasp a cup of coffee that was located in a particular spot on our desk, even minutes later. In one sense these actions are visually guided, even though the visual information is no longer present. But these movements are quite different from the smooth and well-calibrated movements we make under direct visual control. This has been studied in the laboratory by having people look at a solid rectangular block (the Efron blocks described in Chapter 2) and then wait for several seconds in the dark before they make a grasping movement. During the delay, the object is removed, and the person is asked to "pantomime" how they *would* have picked it up (see Figure 7.2). These pantomimed movements are slower, less accurate, and somewhat stylized: not surprisingly, given that the person is *showing* you how to do something rather than actually doing it. This change in

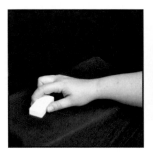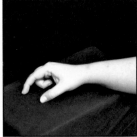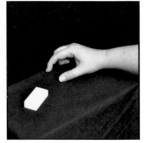

Figure 7.2 In normal grasping, we reach out and pick up the object we see in front of us. In "pantomimed" grasping, we see the object but then it is taken away. After a few seconds' delay, we then reach out and pretend to pick it up. Grasping an object that we can see engages the automatic visuomotor systems in the dorsal stream, whereas pantomimed grasping requires that we use a conscious visual memory of what we saw earlier—a memory that was constructed by the ventral stream.

the character of the movement is present even after a delay as short as two seconds. Of course the person will still open the hand grip more widely for larger than for smaller objects, just as when making real grasps, though they generally do so later in the movement. The hand tends to open less widely during pantomimed grasps than during real grasps—probably because people do not realize that the hand opens much wider than the width of the target object during real grasping movements (see Chapter 2, Figure 2.7).

In contrast to the unrealistic efforts that most of us can make, mime artists can produce very convincing movements to imaginary objects—and indeed convey a whole story by doing so. They can almost convince us that they are climbing a ladder, washing a window, picking up a heavy object, or peeling a banana, just by making movements in mid-air. They do this by first studying closely how such movements are actually made—and exaggerating certain aspects and not others. But the important thing is that while it takes no special skill to pick up a real coffee cup, it requires the well-practiced skill of a mime artist to perform that very same action convincingly when the cup is imaginary (and as we discuss in Box 7.2, stage magicians are adept in a different form of pantomiming). Moreover, unlike the mime artist, we pick real things up without thinking about the details of the object or the movement. It is only when we have to perform an action offline that we have any difficulty.

BOX 7.2 SLEIGHT OF HAND

Professional magicians are adept at doing one thing while pretending to do another. They fool us because their fake actions so closely resemble real ones, while at the same time they distract attention from what they really are doing. For example, in a classic "French drop," magicians make a coin "disappear" by concealing it in one hand rather than transferring it to the other, thereby making a simulated rather than a real grasping action.

Most of us are poor at faking actions in this way. Detailed studies have shown that when pretending to pick up objects that are not really there (pantomimed actions), we move and shape our hands quite differently from when grasping real ones. For example, when we make real grasps our hand normally opens much wider than the size of the object during the course of the reach ("grip overshoot"), whereas this happens much less when we make pantomimed actions. In a recent study, Cristiana Cavina-Pratesi and Gustav Kuhn (who is an accomplished semi-professional magician himself) tested whether, despite their skill, professional magicians might still show such detectable differences between grasping actions made toward real versus imagined objects. In this experiment, when the object was visible (but displaced) during the action, the magicians made pantomimed actions that closely resembled real grasps. The diagram shown in this box plots how wide a margin the magicians and untrained volunteers adopted while opening their hand during reaching. Pretending to reach out and grasp an

(Continued)

object in thin air is shown in light gray, while real grasping of the object is shown in dark gray. Clearly the magicians don't make the mistake of opening their hand too little when pantomiming, providing they can see the object elsewhere on the table (A). However when they were asked to make pantomimed actions when the object was absent (i.e. the object had been taken away), they performed just the same as non-magicians, making the normal mistake of not opening the hand widely (B).

One possibility is that although the visuomotor systems of the dorsal stream are designed to guide actions made directly toward a goal object, prolonged practice can render those systems able to calibrate actions based on visual inputs displaced from the real endpoint of the action as well.

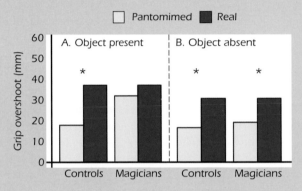

REFERENCE

Cavina-Pratesi, C., Kuhn, G., Ietswaart, M., and Milner, A.D. (2011). The magic grasp: motor expertise in deception. *PLoS ONE*, 6(2), e16568.

When student volunteers in a lab experiment pretend to pick up a block after a two-second delay, they are undoubtedly using a similar strategy to that of the mime artist, but without the mime artist's practiced eye for detail. They are presumably bringing to mind the visual appearance of the object they are pretending to grasp, though in this case only shortly after seeing it. Of course the person has to have perceived the object in the first place, so as to have the information to hold in memory. But as we have argued throughout this book, such perceptual processing is not at all what we use to program and control a normal online grasping movement. It is only in the artificial case of pretending to grasp an object that we need to rely on stored information derived from our perception of that object. So what would happen if a person had no perception of the object's shape and dimensions in the first place? Would that mean that they could not perform the pantomiming grasping task at all?

The reader will remember that our patient Dee Fletcher, who cannot perceive the form and dimensions of objects, still shows excellent scaling of her grasp when she reaches out to pick up objects in real time. To do this, she must be relying entirely on her visuomotor system, since she has no access to relevant perceptual information about the object. Yet despite this excellent online ability, if our argument is correct, Dee should have great difficulty when asked to perform pantomimed grasping of those same blocks. Now, of course, she could no longer rely on her visuomotor system—its visual information would have decayed before she could use it. But nor could she use her perceptual system as a healthy person would, since that is profoundly disabled. Dee would not be able to recall the dimensions of the block she was shown two seconds earlier, because she wouldn't have had a perceptual experience of those dimensions in the first place.

Dee behaves just as these arguments would predict. Her attempts to pantomime the act of picking up the different blocks show little or no relationship to their actual size (see Figure 7.3). Evidently, Dee has no perceptually coded information about the block she just saw that could serve to guide her movements—even though only two seconds have elapsed between last seeing the block and initiating her grasp. It is not that she cannot pretend to grasp the blocks. She goes through the motions, but her attempts bear little resemblance to the actual dimensions of the object shown to her. In fact as we mentioned in Chapter 2, she has no problem making pantomimed

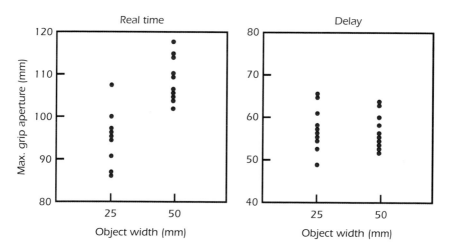

Figure 7.3 Dee's real-time and delayed grasping. Each dot represents her maximum grip aperture on a single grasping trial. When Dee reaches out to grasp objects in real time, her maximum grip aperture scales nicely to the width of the object. In contrast, when she reaches after a two-second delay, when the object is no longer visible, her grip aperture shows no relationship to the width of the object.

actions that do not depend on recent visual experience, but which are based instead on memories of objects long familiar to her. If asked to imagine an everyday thing like a grapefruit or a hazelnut, she can reach out and pretend to pick it up, opening up her grip just like you or I would—large for the grapefruit and small for the hazelnut.

In other words, then, Dee has a problem in dealing with visual shape information that is no longer present in her visual field. When the visual information is still present, she can use her visuomotor system as efficiently as anyone else. It is only when the task we give her requires the use of memory for recently perceived events that her performance falls apart. As we have already argued, since Dee's perception of the location and geometry of objects is compromised, she has no information to store in memory and as a consequence no information on which to base a pantomimed action. Interestingly, Thomas Schenk has recently tested Dee using a mirror set-up where she had to "grasp" in thin air an object that looked as if it was physically real. As in other kinds of pantomiming, however, she performed very poorly. So not only does she need to be able to "see" an object when grasping it, the object needs to actually be there, in tangible reality, and not just *appear* to be there. Yet as Rob Whitwell recently demonstrated in our laboratory, the grasped object doesn't have to be the same size as the one that Dee sees: so long as there's *something* there she still scales her handgrip accurately to what she sees. These are interesting discoveries, and suggest that for the dorsal stream to be engaged and visually guide an action, a full view of the target object is not enough—the action has to have a tactile endpoint of some kind as well.

As an aside here, the reader may recall that the phenomenon of "blindsight" (see Chapter 6) can to a large extent be regarded as "vision without the ventral stream"—albeit resulting from a more "downstream" locus of brain damage than Dee's. We would therefore predict that any blindsight patient whose attempted grasps of a target in their "blind" visual field showed a reliable calibration of grip-size would be subject to same temporal constraints as Dee. That is, their successful grip scaling in the blind field should disappear when required to make a pantomimed grasp after a delay. Precisely this predicted result has been found in the blindsight patient, Susan James, whom we introduced in Chapter 6. In addition, the other blindsight patient we tested, who could avoid unseen obstacles in his blind field when reaching in real time, was unable to do so when a brief delay was introduced between seeing the display and making the reach—and instead behaved as if the obstacle was not there. All this work on Dee and the blindsight patients shows that we need to have access to a functioning ventral stream in order to form the memories that allow us to make a delayed response after the visual information is no longer available.

But what about patients who have the opposite pattern of brain damage to Dee's, in other words patients with dorsal stream damage? What would they do in the pantomime task? Such patients are unable to use vision effectively to control their actions in the here and now, as we saw in patients with optic ataxia (see Chapter 3). We would make the paradoxical prediction, however, that their performance should *improve* if they were forced to refrain from responding to the target, and instead to make a pantomimed movement a few seconds later. After all, their perception of the world is relatively spared, so that during the imposed delay they would be able to invoke their perceptual memory of the target to help them calibrate their response. In other words, they should do *better* after a delay than they would if they responded to the target immediately. This prediction has been borne out in tests of both delayed pointing and delayed pantomime grasping.

In collaboration with Marc Jeannerod and his colleague François Michel, we tested Anne Thiérry, the patient we introduced in Chapter 3 who had developed optic ataxia following damage to both of her parietal lobes. The defining symptom of optic ataxia, of course, is that the patient is unable to make accurate reaching movements toward a visual target. Anne is no exception to this. When we tested her ability to point to briefly flashed spots of light she made big errors, often ending up several centimeters away from the target. But remarkably she made much smaller errors when asked to delay for five seconds after the light spot had gone off before making her pointing attempts. This really is a surprising result, because healthy subjects *never* do better when asked to delay before pointing. In fact, they almost always do worse.

It is very difficult to explain Anne's improvement, except by assuming that she is able to use a quite different system—one that is still relatively intact—to perform the delay task. This spared system, we argue, is her perceptual system, which is not designed to guide immediate responses but does become useful when the response has to be pantomimed. When Anne responds in real time, her faulty visuomotor system leads inevitably to errors in performance. When she has to wait, however, her preserved perceptual system can be used just as it is in healthy people performing the same task, and so she does much better. In other words, despite Anne's extensive brain damage, her relatively intact perceptual system can still permit a visual memory of the light's location to be stored. This visual memory can presumably then guide her successful pantomimed responses. One wonders how much Anne's everyday activities could be improved by training her to slow down and wait before performing an action.

More recently, along with Yves Rossetti and Chris Dijkerman, we have tested the younger patient Irène Guitton, who like Anne suffers from optic ataxia following damage to both parietal lobes, but who unlike Anne shows little sign of other aspects of Bálint's syndrome. Irène's pointing improved when she was forced to delay doing it, just like Anne's. Not only that, we found that her grasping improved after a delay as well when she could not longer see the object and had to pantomime the grasping movement (see Figure 7.4). In other words, she scales her grip better when pantomiming than when simply grasping an object placed in front of her—the exact opposite of Dee Fletcher. These complementary results from Dee and Irène provide a convincing package. They mean that Irène shows a direct double dissociation with Dee between immediate and delayed grasping—she gets better after a delay, while Dee of course gets much worse.

All these experiments on delayed responding make the point that the dorsal (action) stream works in real time and stores the required visuomotor coordinates only for a very brief period—at most for a few hundred milliseconds. The modus operandi appears to be "use it, or lose it." The ventral (perception) stream, on the other hand, is designed to operate over a much longer timescale. For example, when we meet someone, we can remember his or her face (though not always his or her name) for days, months, and even years. This difference in timescale is a reflection of the different jobs the two streams are designed to do. But the difference in timescale is not the only distinction between the dorsal and ventral streams. As discussed at the beginning of this chapter, the two streams actually "see" the world in different ways, using quite different frames of reference.

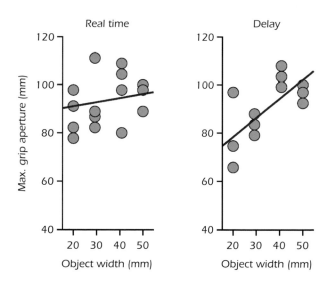

Figure 7.4 In sharp contrast to Dee's performance shown in Figure 7.3, Irène shows an improvement in her grip scaling when tested after a short delay in which she had to pantomime the movement to the object that was no longer visible.

Scene-based versus egocentric frames of reference

When we perceive the size, location, orientation, and geometry of an object, we implicitly do so in relation to other objects in the scene we are looking at. In contrast, when we reach out to grab that same object, our brain needs to focus on the object itself and its relationship to us—most particularly, to our hand—without taking account of the visual context, that is, the scene in which the object is embedded. To put it a different way, perception uses a scene-based frame of reference while the visual control of action uses egocentric frames of reference.

A scene-based frame of reference makes sense for perception because it allows the brain to use all kinds of information to identify objects and their relationships, and then to piece together the meaning of the scene. The job of perception, after all, is to construct a useful internal model or representation of the real world outside. This representation can then serve as a visual foundation for our mental life, allowing us to make inferences about objects in the world and their causal relations, and to decide between different courses of action based on this knowledge.

The use of scene-based metrics means that the brain can construct this representation in great detail without having to compute the absolute size, distance, and geometry of each object in the scene. To register the absolute metrics of the entire scene would in fact be computationally impossible, given the rapidity with which the pattern of light changes on our retina. It is far more economical for perception to compute just the relational metrics of the scene, and even these computations do not generally need to be precise. It is this reliance on scene-based frames of reference that lets us watch the same scene unfold on a small television or on a gigantic movie screen without being confused by the differences in scale.

When we look at something in the world, we cannot help being influenced by the scene that surrounds it. We are obliged to see some things as closer or further away than others, and some things as smaller or larger. The contrast in size between objects is a constantly familiar experience in our perceptual life. For example, when we see an average-size person standing next to a professional basketball player, that person suddenly appears far smaller than they really are. Of course when we get more information by seeing more of the scene, then the true sizes of the two become clearer. Size contrast is perceptual in nature and not a trick of optics. It depends on assumptions that our brain makes about the sizes of objects. For example, our brain, on the basis of previous experience, "knows" that houses are always bigger than people. Film versions of *Gulliver's Travels* make use of this by filming the same actor against artificially small- or large-scale backgrounds. Even though we know it is the same actor, we cannot help but see him as a giant in one case and as a miniature human in the other.

But as we noted earlier, scene-based metrics are the very opposite of what you need when you act upon the world. It is not enough to know that an object you wish to pick up is bigger or closer than a neighboring object. To program your reach and scale your grasp, your brain needs to compute the size and distance of the object in relation to your hand. It needs to use absolute metrics set within an egocentric frame of reference. It would be a nuisance, and potentially disastrous, if the illusions of size or distance that are a normal part of perception were to intrude into the visual control of your movements.

If there really is a difference between the frames of reference used by perception and action systems, it should be possible to demonstrate this in the laboratory. The advent of virtual reality displays, where the experimenter has exquisite control over the way in which objects are presented to the observers, has made this kind of experiment a practical possibility (see Figure 7.5). Artificial "objects" of different

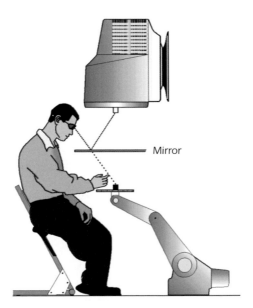

Figure 7.5 The virtual workbench. The observer sees the image of what is on the computer monitor by looking at a mirror while wearing special glasses that make the image three-dimensional. The object depicted on the computer monitor appears to be located below the mirror. When the person reaches out to grasp this virtual object, his hand encounters a real object whose position coincides exactly with what he sees, giving the impression that he is grasping the object shown on the computer screen. The computer and robot arm controlling the position of the real object are linked so that every time the virtual object is placed at a new location the real one moves accordingly. Reproduced from Y. Hu and M.A. Goodale Grasping after a delay shifts, size-scaling from absolute to relative metrics, *Journal of Cognitive Neuroscience*, *12:5* (September, 2000), pp. 856–868, Figure 2. © 2000 by the Massachusetts Institute of Technology, with permission.

sizes can be created and shown to the observer without the possibility of familiarity with particular real objects obscuring the interpretation of the experimental results. In addition it is a simple matter to control the precise period for which the virtual object is visible on the screen.

Using this technique, together with Yaoping Hu, an engineering student working in our lab at the time, we carried out an experiment in which we showed undergraduate volunteers a series of three-dimensional virtual images of target blocks, each of which was paired with an image of another block that was always either ten percent wider or ten percent narrower than the target block. The blocks were never visible for more than half a second. The target blocks were marked with a red spot. Just as in our previous studies with brain-damaged patients, each student was asked to do one of two things. The student either had to reach out and grasp the target block using the index finger and thumb, or to indicate manually the size of the same block using the same finger and thumb. To ensure a natural (not a pantomimed) grasp, the display was designed so that there was a real but unseen block in the same location as the virtual target.

The reason for having two objects, a companion block as well as the target block, was to induce a "size-contrast effect" (see Figure 7.6). It was anticipated that the observer's perception of the target's size would be unavoidably influenced by the presence of a larger or smaller companion. This is exactly what happened. The students consistently judged a target block paired with a large companion as smaller than the same target when it was paired with a small companion. In contrast, when they reached out to *grasp* the target object, they opened their hand to an identical degree whichever companion it was paired with. In other words, the scaling of grip size to the size of the target block was not at all subject to the size-contrast effect that was so compelling during perceptual judgments.

This result is an instructive one. It confirms that the scene-based coding of size that is such a ubiquitous feature of our perceptual experience does not apply at all to the visual coding of size that is used to guide the action of grasping. Of course, it makes good sense to have a visuomotor system that works with real size rather than relative size, so it shouldn't be so surprising that the system is immune to the size-contrast effect. Nonetheless, we can see here a graphic example of our actions being controlled by visual information that is clearly different from our conscious visual experience.

The calibration of grasp does fall victim to the size-contrast illusion, however, when a delay is inserted between viewing the objects and initiating the grasp movement. When the students had to wait for five seconds before picking up the target object that they had just seen, the scaling of their grasp now fell prey to the influence of the companion block. Just as they did when they made perceptual judgments, they

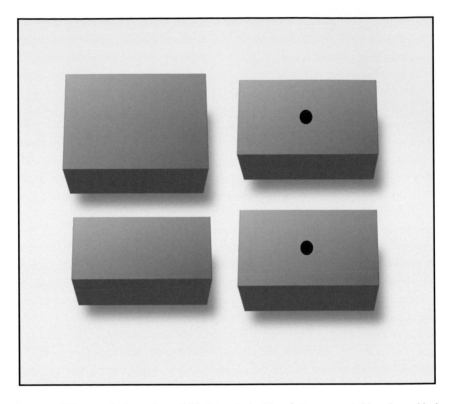

Figure 7.6 When you look at a "target" block (marked with a dot) accompanied by a larger block, it looks slightly smaller than when you see it accompanied by a smaller one. When you reach out to grasp the block, however, your hand opens in flight to match the real size of the target block irrespective of the size of its companion. In short, perception is affected by the contrast in size, but the visual control of action is not.

opened their hand wider when the target block was accompanied by a small block than when it was accompanied by a large block. This intrusion of the size-contrast effect into grip scaling *after a delay* is exactly what we had predicted. Since the dedicated visuomotor systems in the dorsal stream operate only in real time, the introduction of a delay disrupts their function. Therefore when a delay is introduced, the calibration of the grasp has to depend on a memory derived from perceptual processing in the ventral stream, and becomes subject to the same size-contrast illusions that perception is prone to.

These size-contrast results dovetail nicely with the observations we made of pantomime grasping made after a delay in our visual agnosia and optic ataxia patients. Dee Fletcher couldn't do the delayed task at all, whereas Anne and Irène's performance actually improved. Dee could do only the immediate task (using her relatively intact dorsal stream), whereas Anne and Irène could not do it well at all (due to their damaged dorsal stream).

BOX 7.3 ARE THERE TWO SEPARATE BRAIN SYSTEMS FOR OTHER SENSE MODALITIES AS WELL?

Given the dramatic findings we have reported so far for the sense of sight, the reader may wonder whether the brain systems that deal with our other senses work in the same kind of way. Perhaps surprisingly, the answer seems to be yes, at least for the sense of touch—there is now growing evidence that the brain processes touch information in two parallel subsystems, rather than in a single multipurpose system. In other words, pretty much like vision.

The somatosensory (touch) system seems to have an organization remarkably similar to that of the visual system, with two distinct representations of the body existing in the brain, one for the guidance of action and the other for perception and memory. This model, proposed by Chris Dijkerman and Edward De Haan, is supported not only by neuroscience evidence, but by the fact that there are somatosensory illusions that fool our perception without fooling actions based on the same form of bodily sensation. Dijkerman and De Haan call the perceptual representation of the body (which is vulnerable to illusions) our "body image" and the metrical representation that guides action our "body schema."

One illusion to which the body image is prone is the so-called "rubber hand illusion." This illusion is induced by having a person rest one of their arms on a table, but hidden from sight, with an artificial arm made of rubber lying alongside it. The experimenter proceeds to stroke the person's arm while simultaneously stroking the artificial arm in full view. The result is that the person gains a strong impression that the stroking sensations are located not where their real arm is really is, but as if shifted in space to where the artificial arm is lying. Yet when tested in a reaching task with the affected arm, they do not make erroneously long or short movements based on where they wrongly sense the starting point of their arm to be. Instead, their actions are guided on the basis of the true location of the arm, independently of their perceptions—presumably on the basis of the veridical body schema.

Another somatosensory illusion can be created by the applying a vibrator to the biceps of one arm of a blindfolded volunteer—the vibration creates an illusory lengthening of the muscle, resulting in a sensation that the elbow is extended away from its true position. As with the rubber hand illusion, again the volunteer is found to make accurate reaches, despite feeling that the starting point of the arm is different from its true location.

There are even reports of brain-damaged individuals who have a somatosensory equivalent of blindsight—Yves Rossetti calls this phenomenon "numbsense." Such patients are able to locate a touch on an arm which has completely lost the conscious sense of touch, by pointing with the other arm while blindfolded. Rossetti reports that his patient was amazed that she could do this. Even more dramatically, considering the effects of delay in the blindsight experiment by Striemer and colleagues (see earlier in this chapter), Rossetti found that this

(Continued)

numbsense ability evaporated to chance guessing when the patient was asked to delay two to three seconds before making her pointing response. It may be then that while the body schema may survive brain damage that disables the body image, it is constantly reinventing itself, with each reinvention having only a transient lifetime before being lost or replaced. Just like the dorsal visual stream.

While the parts of the brain that hold these representations of the body are less clearly-defined than the two streams within the visual system, it must be no coincidence that they substantially overlap the two visual streams. Both the visual streams contain sub-areas that are "bimodal" (sometimes multimodal)—specifically they can be activated by tactile as well as by visual inputs. Area LO, for example, which we saw earlier is defined in functional neuroimaging experiments by contrasting the brain activation patterns elicited by seeing whole objects versus fragmented versions of those objects, turns out to be activated also when people are given objects to distinguish by hand, out of sight.

There is recent evidence to suggest that the auditory system too may be divided into perception and action pathways. Steve Lomber, a researcher working at the University of Western Ontario, has recently shown that when one region of auditory cortex in the cat is temporarily inactivated by local cooling, the cat has no problem turning its head and body toward the sounds but cannot recognize differences in the patterns of those sounds, whereas when another quite separate area is cooled the cat can tell the sound patterns apart but can no longer turn towards them. These findings in the auditory system—and the work discussed earlier on the organization of the somatosensory system—suggest that a division of labor between perceiving objects and acting on them could be a ubiquitous feature of sensory systems in the mammalian cerebral cortex.

REFERENCES

Dijkerman, H.C. and De Haan, E.H. (2007). Somatosensory processes subserving perception and action. *Behavioral and Brain Sciences, 30,* 189–201.

Lomber, S.G. and Malhotra, S. (2008) Double dissociation of "what" and "where" processing in auditory cortex. *Nature Neuroscience, 11,* 609–616.

Summary

Visual processing in perception and action are very different. They differ in their time constants: very short for action, indefinitely long for perception. The two systems also differ in their metrics: one is scene-based and relational, the other is viewpoint-dependent and uses real-world metrics. And one system is knowledge based and top-down, while the other works from the optic array using first principles, in a bottom-up way. Thus, size-contrast illusions, which by definition affect our perceptual judgments, do not affect our immediate visually guided actions. The experiment on the size-contrast illusion that we discussed in this chapter is only one example in what is now a large field of research looking at the differential effects of illusions on perceptual judgments and visuomotor control. As we shall see in Chapter 8, the experiments on illusions make it clear that the systems in the dorsal stream controlling actions deal with incoming visual information in a very different way from the perceptual systems in the ventral stream. Moreover the same logic applies, to some extent at least, in sense modalities other than vision, particularly touch (see Box 7.3). The sense of hearing does not have the same sensorimotor immediacy as vision or touch, and so the need for a perception/action separation in the brain is less pressing. Nevertheless hearing can act surprisingly well as a substitute for other senses (see Box 7.4).

BOX 7.4 ECHOLOCATION: NOT ONLY BATS DO IT

Everybody has heard about echolocation in bats and dolphins. These creatures emit bursts of sounds and listen to the echoes that bounce back to detect objects in their environment. What is less well known is that people can echolocate, too. A number of blind people have learned to make clicks with their mouths and to use the returning echoes from those clicks to sense their surroundings. Some of these people are so adept at echolocation that they can use this skill to go mountain biking, play basketball, and even navigate unknown environments.

Together with our colleagues, Lore Thaler (now at Durham University in the UK) and Steve Arnott (now at the Rotman Research Institute in Toronto, Canada), we showed that blind experts in echolocation use what is normally the "visual" part of their brain to process the clicks and echoes. To find out how they were doing this, we first made recordings of the clicks and their very faint echoes using tiny microphones in the ears of the blind echolocators as they stood outside and tried to identify different objects such as a car, a flag pole, and a tree. We then played the recorded sounds back to the echolocators while their brain activity was being measured with an fMRI brain scanner.

Remarkably, when the echolocation recordings were played back to the blind experts, not only did they perceive the objects based on the echoes, but they also showed activity in primary "visual" cortex (V1). This activation (shown within the white ellipse on the "inflated" brain in the figure in this box) was particularly striking in one blind echolocator who had lost his vision early in life. Most interestingly, the brain areas that process auditory information (located within the purple ellipse) were no more activated by sound recordings of outdoor scenes containing echoes than they were by sound recordings of outdoor scenes with the echoes removed. Only "visual" cortex showed differential activation to the faint echoes. Importantly, when the same experiment was carried out with sighted people who could not echolocate, these individuals could not make sense of the clicks and echoes, and neither did their brains show any echo-related activity.

(Continued)

141

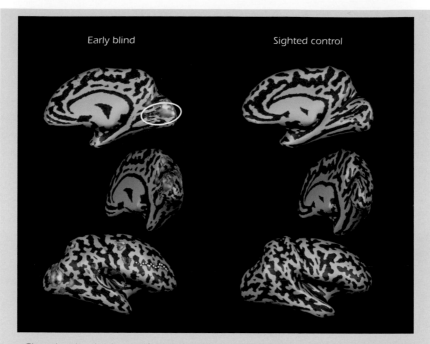

Given that the visual areas of the brain are recruited by the echolocation system, it is perhaps not surprising that experienced blind echolocators appear to use their abilities in a way that seems uncannily similar to vision. Indeed, echolocation provides these individuals with a high degree of independence and self-reliance in their daily life. This has broad practical implications: echolocation is a trainable skill that can potentially offer powerful and liberating opportunities for blind and other visually-impaired people.

What remains a mystery is the reason why what would normally be visual cortex is recruited by the auditory system for echolocation. Is it because it is vacant territory there for the taking or does the inherently topographic nature of this part of cortex (see Chapter 4, Box 4.3) lend itself to the interpretation of the spatial information contained within the echo signals? These are important questions that need to be addressed in future research. Also it is not clear yet whether or not the echolocation system in the blind brain is organized into specialized pathways for the identifying objects on the one hand and spatial navigation and motor control on the other. Nevertheless, it is tantalizing to think there could be an echolocation-for-perception pathway and an echolocation-for-action pathway.

REFERENCE

Thaler, L, Arnott, S.R., and Goodale, M.A. (2011). Neural correlates of natural human echolocation in early and late blind echolocation experts. *PLoS ONE, 6(5)*, e20162.

Further reading

The late Keith Humphrey was instrumental in showing how the distinction between vision for perception and vision for action could help bridge the gap between previous theoretical accounts by individuals like James J. Gibson, David Marr, Richard Gregory, and Ulrich Neisser. Some of these ideas are set out in the following paper:

Goodale, M.A. and Humphrey, G.K. (1998). The objects of action and perception. *Cognition*, 67, 181–207.

For a technical discussion of the computations underlying the visual control of action, see the following paper:

Goodale, M.A., Westwood, D.A., and Milner, A.D. (2004). Two distinct modes of control for object-directed action. *Progress in Brain Research*, 144, 131–144.

VIII

How do the two systems work?

Visual illusions

The size-contrast effect we discussed in Chapter 7 is an everyday occurrence—you do not need to arrange things in any special or artificial way to see it. Simply standing beside a very tall person can make you appear shorter than you really are. But there are many other ways in which our eyes can be fooled, particularly in the contrived scenarios that give rise to the best known visual illusions. No undergraduate course in psychology would be complete without a session devoted to these illusions. We never fail to be impressed with the fact that our eyes can deceive us so thoroughly—and even when the trick is explained we continue to perceive apparent differences in size, orientation, movement, and distance that we know are not really there. Yet many visual scientists would agree with the late Richard Gregory, who argued persuasively that illusions are not just curiosities, but can provide important insights into how the brain constructs our percepts of the world.

One major class of visual illusions depends on so-called pictorial cues—the kinds of cues that are commonly exploited by painters to create a realistic three-dimensional world on a two-dimensional canvas (see Box 8.1). The artist's manipulation of cues like perspective and relative size can create powerful illusions of depth and scale, taking advantage of the way in which our brains carry out an obligatory analysis of the visual scene that confronts us. Such cues provide a major source of information used by the perceptual system to construct our representations of the world. One particular example will illustrate this well. The central circles in the top

BOX 8.1 PICTORIAL CUES TO DEPTH AND SCALE

For centuries, painters have exploited the cues that our perceptual system uses all the time to let it reach plausible interpretations of the ambiguous retinal information it receives. For example, in the real world, objects that occlude our view of other objects in the scene must be closer to us than the occluded objects. In the famous engraving by Albrecht Dürer (1471–1528) shown in this box, the table occludes part of St Jerome and thus is seen as nearer. More distant objects in general are located higher in our visual field than nearby ones. Thus the lion, which is located lower down in the scene is perceived as being closer. Familiar size is also useful. Our knowledge of the real size of lions and people gives a strong indication of their relative position in the scene depicted in this engraving. Moreover, our knowledge of these familiar objects gives information about the size of other less familiar objects that are nearby. Geometric perspective, of course, is a particularly powerful and frequently used cue to distance—and this cue is exploited to good effect in Dürer's engraving. The tricks that artists use to convey depth and scale in pictures are as powerful as they are because they reflect the processes we rely on all the time to perceive the real world.

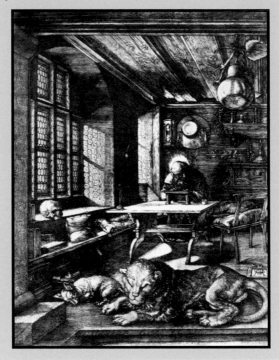

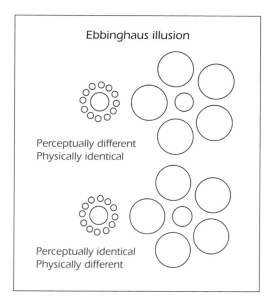

Figure 8.1 In the Ebbinghaus illusion, shown here, the two middle circles in the top two arrays appear to be different in size even though they are actually physically identical. The two middle circles in the bottom display appear to be identical but their real size is actually different. (To convince yourself of this, view each display through a piece of paper with two holes cut in it that reveal only the two central circles.)

two patterns shown in Figure 8.1 are actually identical in size—but it is very hard to resist the impression that the one on the left (surrounded by small circles) is larger than the one on the right (surrounded by larger circles). We can neutralize the illusion by increasing the size of the central circle surrounded by larger circles, as shown in the lower part of Figure 8.1. In this case, although the two central circles look alike, they are actually quite different in size.

A number of explanations have been put forward to account for this illusion, which was first described in the late 19th century by the German psychologist Hermann Ebbinghaus. The most commonly accepted one goes something like this: The brain cannot help but "assume" that the array of smaller circles represents a cluster of objects more distant than the array of larger circles. This remains true even though each cluster includes an object (the central circle) that is different in size from the majority. So the central circle within the array of smaller circles will be perceived as more distant than the one within the array of larger circles. Since the two central circles are actually identical in size as far as the retina is concerned, the perceptual system "infers" that the one that appears to be further away must be the larger of the two. To use a term we will enlarge on later in this chapter, the fact that one central circle looks bigger than the other is a consequence of the perceptual system's attempt to maintain "size constancy" across the entire visual array. That is, the perceptual system attempts to represent the true ("constant") size of objects rather than their retinal size, and it does so by allowing for their apparent distance from the eye.

The brain uses heuristics like this all the time, exploiting the relations between objects in the visual array in order to optimize the perceptual process. In fact, the perceptual system appears to be quite literally unable to avoid making comparisons between different elements in a scene. As a consequence, the system is vulnerable to the kinds of illusory displays devised by Ebbinghaus and many others. Even though you know full well that you are looking at an illusion, you cannot resist it: your beliefs are over-ruled by your perception. These distortions have little practical significance for our everyday perception of the world—their rare occurrences are far outweighed by the usefulness of the scene-based heuristics that cause them. But of course as soon as you *act* on the world, such distortions could lead to problems. Imagine the mishaps that could occur if some accidental conjunction of objects in the visual field created an illusion of size or distance that not only fooled your perception but also your visuomotor control. But as we have already seen, the visuomotor system is largely isolated from perception. Its modus operandi seems to be to disregard information from much of the scene when guiding goal-directed movements like grasping, restricting itself to the critical visual information that is required for that movement. Indeed, we would expect that actions would be immune to the effects of many (but, as we shall see, not all) visual illusions. To test this prediction, we devised, in collaboration with Salvatore Aglioti, an Italian scientist visiting our lab, a new version of the Ebbinghaus illusion. We used solid disks, rather like poker chips, as the central circles, and displayed them against the classic Ebbinghaus background. The set-up is illustrated in Figure 8.2.

Now we could not only test people's perception of the sizes of the disks, but we could also see whether or not the scaling of their grasp was affected by the illusion. The volunteers we tested showed robust perceptual illusions—even in a matching task in which they opened their index finger and thumb to match the perceived diameter of one of the disks. Yet when they reached out to pick up the disk, the size of their grip as they moved toward the disk completely resisted the illusion and was instead tailored to the real size of the disk (see Figure 8.3). Since we first carried out this experiment over fifteen years ago, several other perceptual illusions have been adapted to test their effects on visually guided action (see Figure 8.4). In nearly all cases, the illusions have been found to have little or no effect on the scaling of grasp or the trajectory of a reaching movement despite having strong effects on perception.

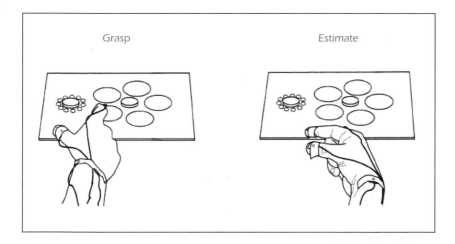

Figure 8.2 A three-dimensional version of the Ebbinghaus illusion. In this experiment, subjects were asked either to reach out and grasp one of the disks, or simply to show us what they thought the size was by opening their finger and thumb a matching amount. On some test trials, the disks were physically identical whereas on other trials they were perceptually identical. Reproduced with permission from A.M. Haffendon and M. Goodale, The effect of pictorial illusion on prehension and perception, *Journal of Cognitive Neuroscience, 10:1*(1998), 122–136, Figure 3, © 1998 by the Massachusetts Institute of Technology.

Nevertheless, it is fair to say that not everyone accepts that grasping is immune to such illusions. Some investigators, notably Volker Franz, a German psychologist, have argued that people attend to the targets quite differently when they are performing an action than they do when they are making an explicit perceptual judgment. Thus, the argument goes, when people reach out to pick up one of the disks in the Ebbinghaus display, they concentrate all their attention on that disk and ignore the other one. But when they are making a perceptual judgment, they cannot avoid comparing one disk with the other. As a consequence, Franz argues, the illusion is always weaker for grasping than for perceptual judgments. In addition, he has pointed out that grip aperture is less sensitive to real changes in target size than are perceptual judgments, and so any effect of the illusion on grasping will always appear to be smaller than its effect on perceptual judgments of size.

These arguments have some validity to them, but there are a number of findings that they cannot explain. For one thing, we showed early on that when the relative sizes of the two disks in the Ebbinghaus display are adjusted so that they appear to be identical, grip aperture continues to reflect their real difference in size. The fact that the illusion affects grasping, but not perception, in this situation cannot be explained by arguing that grasping is less sensitive to changes in size than

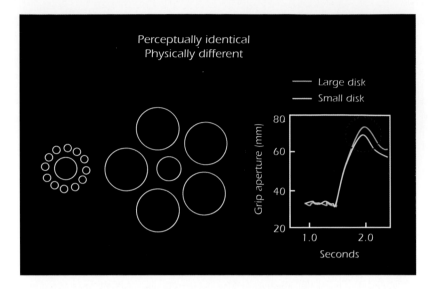

Figure 8.3 A graph showing the changing distance between the finger and thumb (grip aperture) as a typical subject reaches out to pick up two disks, one of which is physically larger than the other. Even though the subject believed that the two disks were the same size, their visuomotor system was not fooled by the illusion. In other words, they scaled their grip aperture to the real size of the objects. Reprinted from *Current Biology*, 5(6), Salvatore Aglioti, Joseph F.X. DeSouza, and Melvyn A. Goodale, Size-contrast illusions deceive the eye but not the hand, pp. 679–685. © (1995), with permission from Elsevier.

perception. Moreover, this difference between grasping and perception was present when people made perceptual estimates of the size of each disk using their finger and thumb—where, just as in the case of grasping, they were attending to only one disk at a time.

But it can still be argued that in all these cases, one is making claims on the basis of the presence of an effect in one case, perception, and the apparent absence of an effect in the other case, action. Volker Franz and others have argued that this could result from differences in the sensitivity of the different measures used in the two cases. To fully rule this out and thereby hammer home the distinction between action and perception, we need a kind of double dissociation—an experiment in which the effect goes one way for grasping and the opposite way for perceptual judgments. This is exactly what was achieved in a recent experiment carried out by Tzvi Ganel in Israel.

Ganel's experiment used a version of the Ponzo illusion (Figure 8.4). This illusion taps into the powerful role that perspective plays in constructing our percepts of depth and distance—and thus the size of objects in the world. Perspective is one of

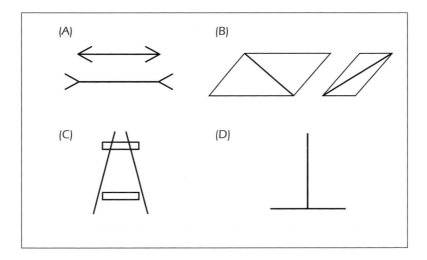

Figure 8.4 Four other pictorial illusions that have been found to have little effect on the visuomotor system. A) The well-known Müller–Lyer illusion. The two lines between the arrowheads appear to be different lengths. B) The Diagonal illusion. The diagonal line in the right-hand figure is actually longer than the diagonal in the left-hand figure. C) The Ponzo (or railway-lines) illusion. In this illusion, the upper bar appears to be longer than the lower bar. D) In the horizontal–vertical illusion the vertical line appears to be longer than the horizontal. When these lines are replaced by solid rods or bars and subjects are asked to pick them up end to end, then although the illusion is still present perceptually, it has little effect on the in-flight scaling of their grasp.

an array of cues that play a critical role in maintaining size constancy—and is often exploited to great effect by artists. The painting shown in Figure 8.5, for example, has been doctored to show just how effective perspective can be in influencing our perception of size. When the couple shown in the distance are transplanted to the foreground they now look very tiny. Ganel took advantage of this cue by presenting his student subjects with two objects of slightly different sizes on a Ponzo illusion background, with the slightly smaller object placed at the diverging end of the display and the larger one at the converging end (see Figure 8.6). In this way, the actually larger object appeared to be the smaller one! In other words, a *real* difference in size was pitted against a *perceived* difference in the opposite direction. He then asked people either to pick up each object by placing their index finger and thumb on the two ends of the object or to estimate its length by opening their index finger and thumb a matching amount.

The results were quite unambiguous. Despite the fact that people believed that the shorter object was the longer one (or vice versa), their grip size reflected the real, not the illusory size of the target objects (see Figure 8.7). Moreover, grip size showed

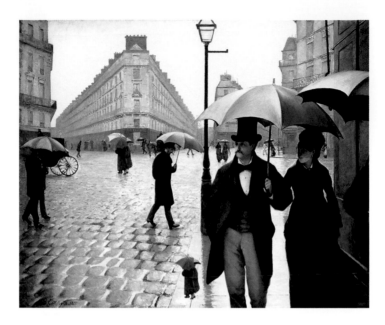

Figure 8.5 This picture of a 19th-century Victorian scene in Paris was painted by Gustave Caillebotte (1848–1894). But what about the two little people down at the front? The picture has been doctored so that they have been copied from further up in the picture. This effect starkly illustrates the importance of pictorial depth cues like perspective in calibrating our perception of size in two-dimensional representations.

the same differential scaling to the real size of the objects whether the objects were shown on the Ponzo display or on a control display in which the background consisted of parallel lines. Yet when people were asked to use their finger and thumb to estimate the size of the target objects rather than pick them up, their estimates reflected the apparent not the real size of the targets (see Figure 8.7). In other words, their grip aperture and their manual estimates went in opposite directions. These results underscore once more a fundamental difference in the way visual information is transformed for action and the way it is transformed for perception. Importantly too, the double dissociation that Ganel observed between grasping and perceptual judgments cannot be explained by arguing, as Franz does, that action and perception are both affected in the same way by illusions, and that the observed differences are simply due to differences in attention between the two tasks or to differences in the sensitivity of the two kinds of measures used.

But yet another, quite different, explanation has been offered for these observed dissociations—even Ganel's double dissociation—between the effects of illusions on grasping and perceptual judgments. This account does not appeal to differences

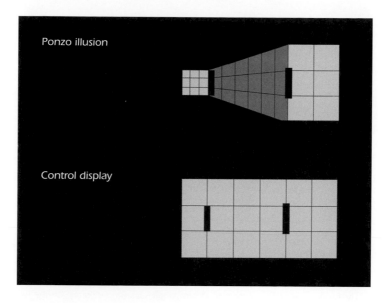

Figure 8.6 Tzvi Ganel's experiment. In the top display, the two objects are placed at opposite ends of a Ponzo illusion background (which, although hard to believe, is actually a flat surface). The object at the converging end of the display is actually physically shorter than the object at the other end, although most people see as looking slightly longer, due to the effects of the Ponzo illusion. The real size of the objects is revealed when they are placed on the rectangular control display shown at the bottom. Reproduced from Tzvi Ganel, Michal Tanzer, and Melvyn A. Goodale, *Psychological Science*, *19*, 221–225, Figure 1. © 2008 by SAGE Publications. Reprinted with permission of SAGE Publications.

in the demands of the task or a failure to equate for possible differences in the size-sensitivity of grip scaling and perceptual judgments. Instead it rests on the idea that the programming of a grasping movement does not depend on computing the *size* of a goal object but on computing the two *locations* on the surface of the object where the grip will be placed. According to the "double-pointing" hypothesis of Jeroen Smeets and Eli Brenner (see Chapter 2, Box 2.1), size is irrelevant to the planning of the trajectories of the finger and thumb, and the apparent scaling of the grip to object size is simply a by-product of the fact that the two digits are heading toward different locations. In other words, we should not be surprised that illusions of size don't affect grasping, they argue, because size is not being used by the brain when we grasp an object. Although, as we saw earlier in Chapter 2 (Box 2.1), Smeets and Brenner's account has been challenged, it has to be acknowledged that their double-pointing hypothesis offers an apparently simple explanation for the lack of an effect of pictorial illusions of size on grasping. Nevertheless, there are a number

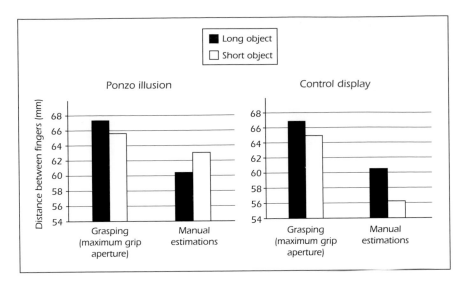

Figure 8.7 The results of Ganel's experiment. When people pick up the objects on the Ponzo background, their maximum grip aperture is scaled to the real difference in size between the two objects. But when asked to estimate their size, they actually estimate the longer object to as being shorter than the other one. In other words, their grip aperture reflects the real difference in size between the two objects, whereas the manual estimates get the sizes reversed. Of course, when the objects are placed on the control display (see Figure 8.6), both the grip aperture and the manual estimates go in the same and correct direction. Reproduced from Tzvi Ganel, Michal Tanzer, and Melvyn A. Goodale, *Psychological Science*, 19, 221–225, Figure 2. © 2008 by SAGE Publications. Reprinted by permission of SAGE Publications.

of other observations of grasping in the context of illusions that cannot easily be accommodated within their account.

First, there is the fact that not all grasps are immune to illusions. Claudia Gonzalez, now based at the University of Lethbridge in Canada, showed that when people reach out and pick up an object using an awkward and unfamiliar grip posture (see Figures 8.8 and 8.9), they are much more likely to show sensitivity to pictorial illusions, such as the Ebbinghaus or Ponzo. (Similar observations have been made when right-handed people use their left hand to pick up objects: see Box 8.2.) We would argue that this sensitivity arises because people show much more conscious and purposeful control over the movements they are making when using an unfamiliar finger posture, directly comparing the posture of their fingers to the size, shape, and location of the goal object. Such deliberate movements are far less likely to engage the "automatic" visuomotor networks in the dorsal stream than a well-practiced and familiar precision grip made with the index finger and thumb. Instead, the control of

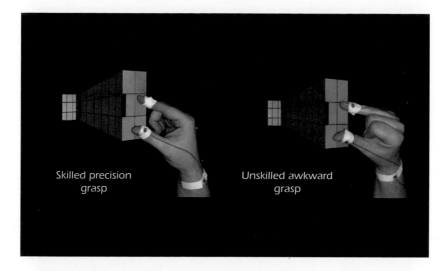

Figure 8.8 Two different kinds of grasp posture used in the experiment by Claudia Gonzalez. On the left is the normal and well-practiced precision grip between forefinger and thumb. On the right is a much more awkward and unfamiliar grip posture where the person uses their thumb and ring finger. In both cases, these grasps are being used to pick up an object placed on a flat Ponzo background (similar to that used in the Ganel experiment). Reprinted from *Neuropsychologia, 46*(2), C.L.R. Gonzalez, T. Ganel, R.L. Whitwell, B. Morrissey, and M.A. Goodale, Practice makes perfect, but only with the right hand: sensitivity to perceptual illusions with awkward grasps decreases with practice in the right but not the left hand, pp. 624–631, Figure 2. © 2008, with permission from Elsevier.

awkward movements is likely to involve perceptual processing in the ventral stream, so that we can monitor our movements consciously. If this reasoning is correct, then as these initially awkward movements become more automatic and natural following practice (so that we no longer monitor them consciously), they should become less sensitive to the effects of the illusory background. In fact, this is exactly what Gonzalez found. After three or four days of practice picking up objects with the initially awkward thumb and ring finger grip, our grip scaling becomes as immune to the illusion as it is when we use the familiar precision grip. Such observations are difficult to reconcile with Smeets and Brenner's double-pointing hypothesis. If the two digits are controlled individually, it shouldn't matter whether the grasping movement is awkward or practiced; in both cases, Smeets and Brenner would predict that the grasp itself would be immune to the illusion.

Second, there is the matter of delay. As we saw in Chapter 7 in the experiments carried out by Yaoping Hu, when even a small delay is introduced between viewing a size-contrast illusion and reaching out to grasp the target object, grip aperture

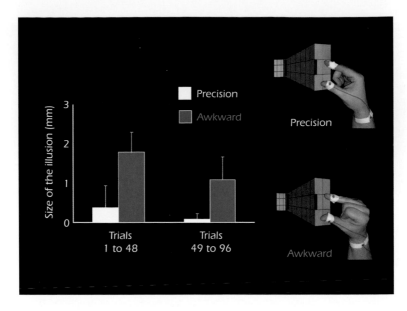

Figure 8.9 As shown in this graph, the scaling of the precision grip is not influenced by the Ponzo illusion. In sharp contrast, the awkward grasp is—and this sensitivity decreases only slightly over the testing session. Reprinted from *Neuropsychologia*, 46(2), C.L.R. Gonzalez, T. Ganel, R.L. Whitwell, B. Morrissey, and M.A. Goodale, Practice makes perfect, but only with the right hand: sensitivity to perceptual illusions with awkward grasps decreases with practice in the right but not the left hand, pp. 624–631, Figure 3. © 2008, with permission from Elsevier.

BOX 8.2 GRASPING ILLUSIONS WITH THE LEFT HAND

Almost all studies that have looked at the effects of pictorial illusions on grasping have studied the scaling of the right-hand grip of right-handed people. But what would happen if people were asked to pick up targets with their less dextrous left hand? This was exactly the question asked by Claudia Gonzalez. She and her colleagues reasoned that if right-handed people used their left hand to pick up a target in the context of a pictorial illusion, such as the Ebbinghaus or Ponzo, they would be much more aware of what they were doing—and would attend much more closely to the way in which their fingers were moving towards the goal object. Because the movements of the left hand were more deliberate and cognitively controlled, they were less likely to engage the "automatic" visuomotor networks in the dorsal stream as thoroughly as movements made with the experienced right hand. As a consequence, Gonzalez argued, perceptual information from the ventral stream would be used to guide the grasping movement—and the grip aperture of the left hand would be scaled to the perceived rather than the real size of the target. This is precisely what she and her colleagues found (see right side of figure in this box which illustrates the effect of the Ponzo and Ebbinghaus illusions on grip scaling in the left and right hand of right-handers).

(Continued)

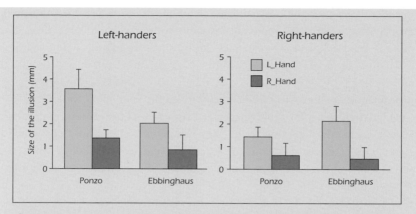

Gonzalez went on to show that, even in left-handers, the left hand is often more sensitive to pictorial illusions than the right hand (see left side of figure). This is because left handedness is usually defined in terms of tool use (i.e. the hand that is used to write with, hammer nails, or wield a knife) rather than the hand that is used to pick something up with a precision grasp. In fact, when Gonzalez measured hand use in a precision grasping task, she found that many left-handers, even strong left-handers, preferred to use their right hand when picking up small objects.

It could be the case that the use of the right hand in a skilled grasping task reflects a property of the brain that is ancient and hard-wired. Support for this idea comes from a series of elegant studies on hand preferences in chimpanzees, our closest phylogenetic relatives. William Hopkins, a primatologist at the Yerkes Primate Laboratory in Atlanta, USA, has found that chimpanzees using a precision grip to grasp small pieces of food are more likely to use their right hand. This population-level hand preference has been observed both in the precision grip and in the so-called "tube task" in which chimpanzees have to extract peanut butter from a tube using the index finger of one hand while holding the tube with the other. Hopkins and his colleagues have also shown that rearing chimpanzees in different environments has no influence on the expression of handedness; instead nature, not nurture, appears to be the key factor. Thus, the right hand "advantage" for visuomotor control might reflect a left-hemisphere specialization that pre-dates the brain asymmetries associated with tool use and language. After all, skilled visually-guided grasping in primates almost certainly emerged before tool use and speech.

REFERENCES

Gonzalez, C.L.R., Ganel, T., Whitwell, R.L., Morrissey, B., and Goodale, M.A. (2008). Practice makes perfect, but only with the right hand: sensitivity to perceptual illusions with awkward grasps decreases with practice in the right but not the left hand. *Neuropsychologia, 46,* 624–631.

Hopkins, W.D. (2006). Chimpanzee right-handedness: internal and external validity in the assessment of hand use. *Cortex, 42,* 90–93.

suddenly becomes affected by the illusion to a quite dramatic degree. Of course this is exactly what we expected—after all, visuomotor control works in real time. When a delay is imposed, perception intrudes. And if our perception is influenced by an illusion, so is the delayed grasping movement. Again, this result doesn't fit with the double-pointing hypothesis—unless one argues that real-time skilled grasping uses independent digit control to specific locations on the goal object, whereas delayed or awkward grasping, for some unspecified reason, uses grip control on the basis of object *size*. But what reason could there be for that? The obvious one would be the use of different visual streams for perception and action. In other words, even if Brenner and Smeets's ideas were correct (and, as we saw in Box 2.1 in Chapter 2, this seems unlikely), this modified double-pointing explanation for immediate and delayed grasping could be readily mapped on to the perception-action duality we have been developing throughout this book.

Are all illusions the same?

We have seen that illusions can fool visually guided movements that are either delayed in time or awkward to make—in both cases because these kinds of consciously controlled actions rely on the perceptual mechanisms in the ventral stream. But there are certain visual illusions to which even skilled actions made in real time are vulnerable. These illusions affect visuomotor control because they arise at an early stage of cortical visual processing, before the visual system splits into two streams. While they provide exceptions to the rule, these illusory effects on action are important, because they force investigators to give more careful consideration to the predictions made by the two-stream model of perception and action.

In collaboration with our late colleague Richard Dyde, we used two different illusions of orientation (see Figure 8.10), both of which induce a strong effect on the perceived tilt of the central vertical line or grating—about 10° on average in both cases. We were able to measure the strength of these illusions by asking observers to adjust a card to match the tilt of the central target in either case. But though similar in strength, the two illusions are actually very different in their causal origin, and this difference gave rise to quite different outcomes when our observers made a response direct toward the central target. When we presented a target centered within a large frame (as shown at the bottom of Figure 8.10), the observers showed no illusion at all when they made a grasping or "posting" action toward the target, just as we saw for size in the Ebbinghaus and Ponzo illusions. Yet when we used the patterns like those shown at the top, our observers' posting movements toward the central grating were shifted by the same average 10° as when they reported their subjective perceptions.

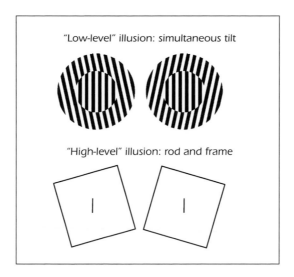

Figure 8.10 The simultaneous "tilt illusion" (top) and the "rod and frame illusion" (bottom). In both illusions we see the stripes or central line to be tilted in opposite directions according the tilt of striped background (top) or the tilt of the frame (bottom). The reasons for this, however, are different for the two illusions. The simultaneous tilt illusion is probably the result of local inhibitory effects within the primary visual cortex, and therefore would be passed on to both visual streams. As a consequence this illusion affects both perception and action. The rod and frame illusion, however, depends on the same kinds of perceptual mechanisms as the pictorial illusions already mentioned, and like those, affects perception but not action.

We had already predicted these different outcomes on the basis of prevailing views in the literature as to how the two illusions work. By all current theoretical accounts, the "rod and frame" illusion (Figure 8.10 bottom) is a context- or scene-based one, and therefore may be assumed to come into play well within the ventral stream itself. The large tilted frame induces a wholesale reorienting of the observer's reference coordinates. This kind of scene-based illusion fully exploits the way the ventral stream works. Yet it should not affect the visuomotor system in the dorsal stream, which does not operate this way at all. In contrast, the simultaneous tilt illusion is believed to be generated within the primary visual cortex (V1) through local interactions between neighboring columns of orientation-coding neurons, well before the anatomical point of divergence between the dorsal and ventral streams. Consequently the distorting effects of this "simultaneous tilt illusion" on the visual signal would be passed on to both visual streams in the brain, thereby misleading both perception and action equally.

Michael Morgan and colleagues at City University in London, UK, have provided a second example. They used the Poggendorff illusion, another illusion believed to be caused by local interactions in early visual cortex. This illusion causes the viewer to see two collinear line segments as misaligned when presented diagonally "behind" a pair of vertical lines (see Figure 8.11). In this experiment the action required was to point to where a line on one side should be extrapolated to intersect with the vertical line on the other side. The pointing responses revealed large errors; if anything bigger than those made during perceptual judgments. Just like the simultaneous tilt illusion, then, the visual miscoding arising in early visual cortex was transmitted to both the visuomotor and the perceptual systems.

The moral of this story is that the best kind of illusion for revealing a dissociation between perception and action is one that is demonstrably "higher-order," in other words, dependent on perceptual/cognitive mechanisms deep in the ventral stream. This is exactly what was done in a recent experiment by Grzegorz Króliczak, a former graduate student in our lab, who used the hollow-face illusion, an illusion clearly of a high level in that it has to depend on top-down influences from our knowledge of faces. Króliczak did this work together with Richard Gregory and Priscilla Heard, who were visiting our lab at the time.

The hollow-face illusion, in which a hollow mask is perceived (incorrectly) as a normal protruding face, has two important characteristics that make it quite different from other illusions that have been used to examine the possible dissociation between perception and action. First, unlike traditional illusions of size or position, it involves a reversal of perceived depth; and second, under the right testing conditions, as Richard Gregory has shown, this depth reversal can "push" the perceived

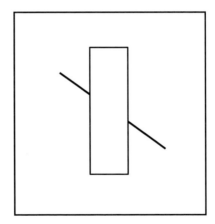

Figure 8.11 The Poggendorff illusion. The diagonal line segments look to be discontinuous, but are actually perfectly aligned. Most probably this illusion arises at an early stage of visual analysis, in area V1, much like the simultaneous tilt illusion shown in Figure 8.10.

front of the face out from its true location by several centimeters. Thus, there should be a dramatic difference between the effect of the hollow-face illusion on perceptual judgments and its effect on visually guided movements. The difference should be much larger than those seen in experiments with other illusions such as the Ponzo or Ebbinghaus, where the differences between the effects on perception and action are typically no more than a few millimeters—which could help to explain why the results have sometimes been hard to replicate clearly.

In Króliczak's study, people used their fingers to make a quick flicking movement at a small target attached to the inside surface of the hollow—but apparently normal—face, or on the surface of a normal convexly protruding face (see Figure 8.12). In other words, they were asked to flick the target off the face as if it were a small insect (an ecologically plausible task). The notion was that the fast flicking would engage the visuomotor networks of the dorsal stream—and thus would be directed to the actual rather than the perceived position of the target. On other occasions, they estimated the perceived position of the target with respect to the background from which the face appeared to protrude. The results were striking. Despite the presence of a robust illusory reversal of depth, with the subjects perceiving the hollow face as if it were a normal protruding face, the flicking movements were well directed to the real, not the illusory location of the target (see Figure 8.13).

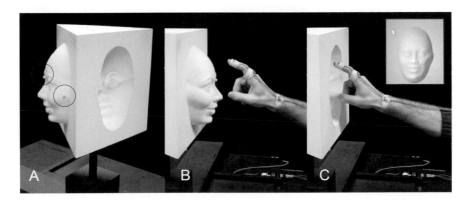

Figure 8.12 The apparatus we used to test perceptual judgments and visuomotor control with the hollow-face illusion. A) Two small magnets (marked with circles) were placed on the cheek and forehead of either the normal face or the hollow mask. B) The fast flicking movement made towards the normal face. C) The same movement made towards the illusory (actually hollow) face. The inset shows a photograph of a bottom-lit hollow face, creating the illusion of a normal convex face. Reprinted from *Brain Research*, *1080*(1), Grzegorz Króliczak, Priscilla Heard, Melvyn A. Goodale, and Richard L. Gregory, Dissociation of perception and action unmasked by the hollow-face illusion, pp. 9–16, Figure 1. © (2006), with permission from Elsevier.

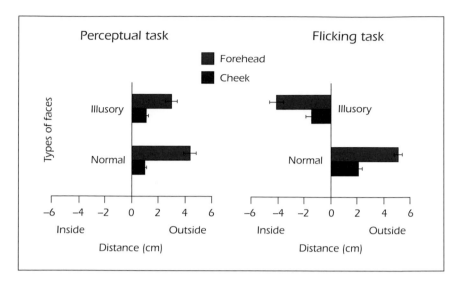

Figure 8.13 Dissociation between perception and action with the hollow-face illusion. In the perceptual task (left-hand graph), the observers were asked to mark (with reference to a line on a piece of paper) the perceived positions of the target on the foreheads and cheeks of the faces. The mean distances of the pencil marks from the line indicating the reference plate (see Figure 8.12) are shown on the horizontal axis. The illusory face (which was actually hollow) appeared to be a normal convex face and so observers saw the targets as sticking out in front just like they did with the normal protruding face. In the action task (right-hand graph), the flicking hand was not fooled by the illusion and went inside the hollow mask. Reprinted from *Brain Research*, *1080*(1), Grzegorz Króliczak, Priscilla Heard, Melvyn A. Goodale, and Richard L. Gregory, Dissociation of perception and action unmasked by the hollow-face illusion, pp. 9–16, Figures 2 and 3. © (2006), with permission from Elsevier.

The results of this experiment show that the visuomotor system in the dorsal stream can guide the finger to the actual locations of targets in the real world, even when perceived positions of those targets are influenced, or even reversed, by processing in the ventral stream that drives the perception of faces.

How does the dorsal stream compute size and distance?

Studies of illusions are not just fun—they also tell us about differences in the underlying mechanisms of depth processing in the two visual streams. In particular, they strongly suggest that the visuomotor system does not use pictorial cues to compute the size and distance of goal objects like the ventral stream. Yet we have to be able to aim and form our grasp accurately toward objects at different distances, so what information is the dorsal stream using to gauge distance? How, for example, does it compute the real size of the target disk presented in an Ebbinghaus illusion, or the real distance of the targets on the hollow but apparently protruding face in the hollow-face illusion? Presumably whatever cues are used, they would have to be reliable and accurate—and certainly not subject to these illusions. In other words, they would have to be independent of the visual context within which the goal object is seen. One way of computing an object's distance (and, as we shall see, its size) takes advantage of the fact that we have two eyes. Because the two eyes each have a different view of the world (technically known as stereopsis) and our brain has information about their degree of convergence (i.e. the slight difference between the eyes' lines of sight), it is possible to compute the real distance of an object we are looking at (see Figure 8.14). Then because the image of the object will have a certain size on the retina, the brain can use this inferred distance information to compute the object's actual size, effectively using simple trigonometry. This kind of computation

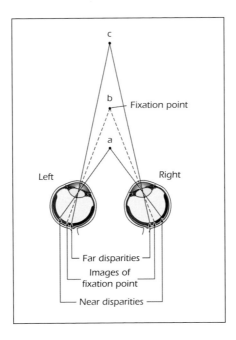

Figure 8.14 When we fix our gaze on an object in the middle distance (b), then that object falls on the same point on our two retinas. However, objects in front of or behind that will fall on non-corresponding points, allowing the brain to compute their distance from the viewer relative to the point of fixation. This powerful cue to depth is called stereopsis. In addition, the extent to which the two eyes are converged on the fixated object gives a measure of its absolute distance from the observer. These two binocular cues to distance (stereopsis and convergence) complement the various pictorial cues discussed earlier.

is highly reliable and will deliver accurate size and distance information independent of the details of any particular scene.

Of course we are all familiar with the power of binocular cues to depth through watching three-dimensional films such as *Avatar*—or looking at pictures in an old-fashioned stereoscope. But although these artificial contrivances give strong, even exaggerated, perceptions of depth, the pictorial cues that are present in one eye's view of the scene already provide irresistible impressions of depth and distance. For example, when we see a painting by one of the old masters, we are highly influenced by the pictorial cues like perspective that are emphasized in the picture, even though we not only know that the picture is flat but we also have binocular information from our two eyes telling us that it is flat (see Box 8.1). Exactly the same argument can be made for two-dimensional TV and movies, in which the images contain no binocular depth information. (As with the paintings, we ignore the binocular depth information that tells us that the screen is in fact flat.) Even when we look at the real world, binocular information makes only a small contribution to our conscious perception of depth. The simple act of covering one eye will reveal that this is true. While there is some reduction in the richness of the percept, the world still looks fully three-dimensional.

Where binocular vision really comes into its own is when we have to act on the world—particularly on objects within arm's reach. Try threading a needle with one eye closed! Experiments have shown that when we reach out to grasp objects under monocular viewing conditions, our movements are much slower, more tentative, and less accurate than the same movements made under normal binocular viewing conditions. It is binocular information (derived from stereopsis and/or monitoring of the convergence angle of the eyes as we look at the goal object) that allows us to make grasping movements that are calibrated correctly for distance and tailored to the real size of the object. So this is why we are able to reach out and accurately flick targets of a hollow-face, even though we see it as a normal protruding face—and why we can scale our grasp to the correct size of a target presented in the context of a Ponzo or Ebbinghaus illusion, even though the target looks larger or smaller than it really is.

Dee Fletcher, because of her visual form agnosia, does not have access to most pictorial cues. Her visuomotor system has to fall back almost entirely upon its normally preferred source of depth information, in other words, on binocular vision. Without binocular vision, her visuomotor system has real problems. When we tested Dee on a grasping task with one eye covered, her grip scaling became surprisingly inaccurate. In fact, she opened her hand wider for a given-size object the closer that object was to her. In the absence of binocular cues, her brain could not compute the real size of the object the way a normal brain would, simply because it could not infer the viewing distance. Without binocular information, she couldn't tell if a given image on her eye represented a large object far away or a small object close up.

What information does the dorsal stream derive from binocular viewing? It could be stereopsis, in that Dee's brain might directly compute viewing distance from a comparison of the different views that each eye receives. But alternatively, it might be that she simply fixates her gaze on the object, and then her brain somehow monitors how much her eyes are converging on it. In fact, this second possibility turns out to be correct. With Mark Mon-Williams and Rob McIntosh, we found that her reaches under binocular conditions when she pointed to targets located at different distances is critically dependent on how much she converges her eyes when looking at the target. We discovered this by artificially making her eyes converge too much or too little, using a wedge prism placed over one of her eyes. She made big errors in the extent of her reaches that could be almost entirely accounted for by the geometry of the prism. In other words, her brain must have been relying very heavily on monitoring her eye convergence in computing how far to reach. Normal observers too are affected by such prisms, but not to anything like the overwhelming extent that Dee is affected. They of course have access to pictorial cues like perspective, which can help them gauge distance—the same cues that imbue paintings with their apparent depth. But because these cues depend on form perception, they are unavailable to Dee.

Although figuring out the required distance for a grasping movement depends more on convergence of the two eyes than it does on stereopsis, the scaling of the grasp and the final placement of the fingers seems to depend more on stereopsis than convergence. Thus, the two binocular cues make separate and quite different contributions to reaching and grasping. But binocular cues are not the only source of information for the control of action. There are other cues, like the motion of the world on our retina when we move, that the system can and does use. When we move around (even when we simply move our head from side to side), near objects in the world move in the opposite direction from more distant ones. This differential motion on the retina is called motion parallax—and it can substitute for the absence of binocular vision, including in Dee. In fact, patients who have lost an eye through accident or disease move their heads a lot when picking up objects, presumably to compensate for the loss of binocular vision. It turns out that motion parallax in both patients and normally-sighted people contributes more to the computation of reach distance than it does to the formation of the grasp. (Parenthetically, the reader may note that the differential contributions that these cues make to the reach and grasp components respectively are much more consistent with Jeannerod's dual-channel hypothesis of the reach-to-grasp movement than they are with Smeets and Brenner's double-pointing account (see Chapter 2, Box 2.1).)

Of course, even when one eye is covered and the head immobilized, healthy people are still able to reach out and grasp objects reasonably well, suggesting that static monocular cues can be used to program and control grasping movements. In fact, together with Jonathan Marotta, we showed that pictorial cues, such as familiar size and how high something is within the visual scene (the further something is away from us, the higher it is in the scene), can be exploited to program and control grasping. Nevertheless, this reliance on pictorial cues occurs only when binocular cues are not available. In other words, binocular information from convergence and/or stereopsis typically overrides the contributions made by pictorial cues.

How does the ventral stream construct our visual world?

At the beginning of Chapter 7, we suggested that the perceptual system uses scene-based coding and relational metrics to construct the rich and detailed representation of the real world that we enjoy. The ultimate reason for having such representations is so that we can use them as a foundation for thinking about past, present, and future visual worlds and for planning our actions. To serve such a generalized function, our memory bank of information about objects in the world has to be in a form that is independent of the particular viewpoint from which the objects were first encountered. That is, the perceptual system has to abstract the invariant aspects of objects, which can then serve, as it were, as *symbols* for what we see in the world. The system has to distance itself from the details of each individual view of the object on the retina. It has to get away from the fact that the projected image of a door on the retina could be rectangular or trapezoidal, according to the viewpoint from which we see it. That instantaneous view may be important for grasping an object, but it is a distraction when what we wish to store is the identity of the object. What we perceive is a rectangular door, though inclined perhaps at a particular angle.

Primitive art and the drawings of young children, paradoxically perhaps, reflect this high-level abstract nature of our perceptual representations. In some sense, children are representing what they "know" rather than what they "see." When children draw a busy scene, all of the objects in the scene—people, cars, houses, and so on—will be in full view (see Figure 8.15). No object will obscure part of another; nor will objects be scaled for viewing distance. Nor do their drawings incorporate perspective to take into account the observer's viewpoint. For an artist to render a "faithful" representation of a scene takes years of training and considerable mental effort. The artist has to *deduce* the perspective projection of a scene on the eye; it is not available to us as a direct perceptual experience. For

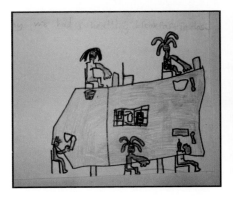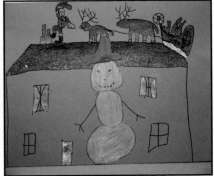

Figure 8.15 The drawing on the left, which was drawn at age six, shows the typical absence of pictorial cues to distance and size in young children's drawings. There is no perspective, no occlusion, and no size scaling with distance. There is, however, relative size scaling (the table is larger than the people) and distance is signaled by the height of objects in the picture (the people at the top are further away). The drawing on the right which was done a year later begins to incorporate some additional pictorial cues including occlusion and size scaling with distance. Reprinted with the kind permission of Ross Milner.

example, returning to the door for a moment, we may see a wide open door or one that is closed—but what we are not aware of is a narrow trapezoid in one case and a wide rectangle in the other. To draw the open or closed door, we have to "work backwards" to reconstruct what instantaneous snapshot would create that perception. In other words, we have to put on the canvas what the light from the scene has put on our retina.

This aspect of perception, in which different projected image shapes are interpreted as being the same object, is called shape constancy. Our visual experience is characterized by a number of these perceptual constancies, which collectively ensure that we recognize a given object pretty much independently of the particular conditions under which we happen to encounter it. Other constancies include color constancy, brightness constancy, and size constancy. So, for example, a blue shirt looks blue both indoors under fluorescent lighting and outdoors in bright sunlight—even though the wavelengths of light hitting the retina under the two conditions are very different. Similarly, a black T-shirt outdoors on a sunny day certainly looks black even though it actually reflects more light into the eye than does a white T-shirt seen indoors. And two identical balls, one viewed close by on a beach and another seen 30 meters away are both perceived as the same size, despite one occupying much more area on the retina than the other. All of these constancy phenomena cooperate to help us interpret the many objects that we may see in a complex scene, and there is a continuous "bootstrapping" process, in which each object provides part of the context for the others.

The boundary between perception and knowledge is not a sharp one. Not only does perception inform knowledge, but also knowledge constantly informs perception. We have all experienced perceptual learning. The novice, whether he is a beginner at microscopy, bird watching, or military surveillance, will literally not see things in the same way as the expert. This use of knowledge to shape our perceptual experience (what we called top-down processing in Chapter 1) is a principle used in many machine recognition systems, such as those designed for recognizing handwritten script. In a real sense, what we "see" in our perceptual experience is determined in large part by what we already know.

Carefully examine the two pictures in Figure 8.16 and the corresponding pictures in Figure 8.17. Can you spot the differences? Pairs of picture like these which have a difference in one quite major feature, have been used to demonstrate "change blindness." When viewing such pictures successively, observers often fail to notice the difference, particularly in pictures like the one showing the two children. The more perceptually salient difference in the picture of the young woman is easier to see, even though it is less physically salient than the difference in the picture of the children.

The influence of previous knowledge on perception has led some theorists to argue that what we experience is a representation of a virtual, not a real, world. What they mean by this is that our knowledge of the world helps us construct a rich and complex experience that is derived as much from memory as it is from visual input. The influence of memory and expectation can be seen in the familiar children's game in which you have to spot the difference between two almost identical pictures. Experimenters like Ron Rensink and Kevin O'Regan have taken this game to new heights. Using modern computer graphics, they have doctored photographs of everyday scenes to generate pairs of pictures that are identical except for one feature. When they show these pairs of pictures on a computer screen one after the other, it takes most people many alternations to spot the difference. In fact some people never do see the difference, until it is pointed out to them. Take a look again at the two pictures of young children shown in Figures 8.16 and 17. Even though the difference between them, once spotted, is obvious, you probably didn't see it immediately. In fact, to find the difference, you may have had to resort to the strategy of carrying out a point-by-point comparison. And if you hadn't been told to look for a difference, you would probably never have seen it. Both pictures convey the same overall meaning or significance—the feature that is different between them is not essential to that meaning. In practice the difference in physical terms can be quite large—but as long as that difference is not relevant to the meaning of the scene, it

168

will typically not be noticed. On the other hand you probably spotted the difference between the two pictures of a young woman also shown in on Figures 8.16 and 8.17 far more quickly. Although the difference is small, it changes our whole percept of the face, and faces are generally the prime targets of our attention, even when a scene contains many other elements.

Film-making again provides wonderful examples of how our expectations determine a good deal of what we see. What is apparently a continuous piece of action is often in fact a compilation of scenes shot at different times that have then been strung together to convey the narrative. The order in which the scenes were actually filmed is often quite different from how they unfold on the screen. It is the job of the continuity editor to make sure that the scenes fit together seamlessly and that, for example, an actor with a moustache at the beginning of a scene is still wearing it at the end. Fortunately for them, they do not have to do this perfectly. They can make big mistakes and still get away with it—particularly when the mistakes they make are not crucial to the narrative. In other words, even if the picture hanging on the wall is present in one scene and missing in the next, most people in the audience will not notice.

Perception, then, is not a passive process, in which we simply experience whatever is on our retina at any one time. It is also more than just a simple process of matching the incoming visual information against stored templates that have been built up from previous experiences. Instead, it seems that much of what we "see" is an internal invention based on plausible assumptions about what is out there in the world. We do not validate these assumptions until we actually look directly at things

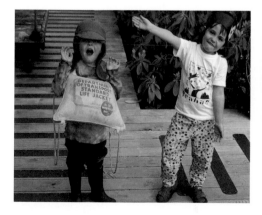 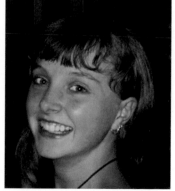

Figure 8.16 Compare the two pictures in this figure with the corresponding pictures in Figure 8.17. Can you spot the differences?

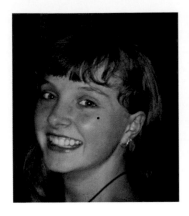 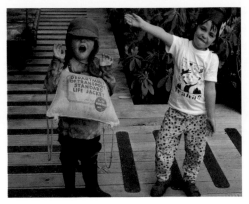

Figure 8.17 Comparison pictures for Figure 8.16. See text.

in our visual environment—yet subjectively we have the impression of a stable and complete world that extends throughout our visual field, rich in detail and meaning. But just as a film set made of painted plywood facades, with the occasional cardboard cactus, may suffice in a Western movie—and is a great deal cheaper to use than filming on location—it seems that we unwittingly make do with secondhand visual experience much of the time in real life as well. It is only when we focus our attention on the relevant part of the visual field that our experience becomes fully informed by what's actually out there in the world.

Further Reading

For an excellent introduction to the psychology of perception, including geometric illusions and the perceptual constancies, the reader might wish to consult:

Gregory, R.L. (1997). *Eye and Brain* (5th edition). Oxford: Oxford University Press.

The following articles examine the evidence that many of our actions are immune to pictorial illusions:

Goodale, M.A. (2008). Action without perception in human vision. *Cognitive Neuropsychology*, *25*, 891–919.

Goodale, M.A. (2011). Transforming vision into action. *Vision Research*, *51*, 1567–1587.

Milner, A.D. and Dyde, R.T. (2003). Why do some perceptual illusions affect visually guided action, when others don't? *Trends in Cognitive Science*, 7, 10–11.

For an incontestable demonstration of the dissociation between perception and action in the context of pictorial illusions, see:

Ganel, T., Tanzer, M., and Goodale, M.A. (2008). A double dissociation between action and perception in the context of visual illusions: opposite effects of real and illusory size. *Psychological Science*, 19, 221–225.

For a discussion of "change blindness" and its implications for understanding our everyday visual experience, see:

Simons D.J. and Rensink, R.A. (2005). Change blindness: past, present, and future. *Trends in Cognitive Neurosciences*, 9, 16–20.

IX

Getting it all together

Throughout this book, we have been advancing the idea that the ventral perception stream and the dorsal action stream are two independent visual systems within the primate cerebral cortex. Nevertheless, the two evolved together and play complementary roles in the control of behavior. In some ways, the limitations of one system are the strengths of the other. The ventral stream delivers a rich and detailed representation of the world, but throws away the detailed metrics of the scene with respect to the observer. In contrast, the dorsal stream delivers accurate metrical information about an object in the required egocentric coordinates for action, but these computations are fleeting and are for the most part limited to the particular goal object that has been selected. Of course somehow the two streams must end up cooperating harmoniously with each other, but the fact that they do so doesn't mean that the distinction between them thereby disappears. After all, to invoke a metaphor used by a neuroscientist colleague, a husband and wife may have utterly different personalities, habits, and ways of working and thinking—but that doesn't mean they cannot live a closely cooperative and harmonious life together.

The constant interplay between the two streams is something that can be seen in almost everything we do. For example, suppose while walking down the street, you recognize an old friend walking toward you, someone that you have not seen for a long time. As the friend draws near, you reach out and shake his outstretched hand. This familiar experience illustrates the different but complementary roles played by the two visual streams in our everyday social behavior. It is your ventral stream, through its intimate connections with long-term memory, that enables you to recognize your friend—and to see the significance of his outstretched hand. But it is your dorsal stream that enables you to grasp his hand successfully. Although it might seem inefficient and even cumbersome to have two specialized visual systems, which then have to be coordinated, this arrangement has some important advantages over a single jack-of-all-trades system.

Putting thought into action

A useful way of understanding the need for two systems, each doing a different job, can be found in robotic engineering. In particular, a neat analogy to the relationship between the two visual streams is provided by *tele-assistance* (see Figure 9.1). Tele-assistance is one of the general schemes that have been devised whereby human

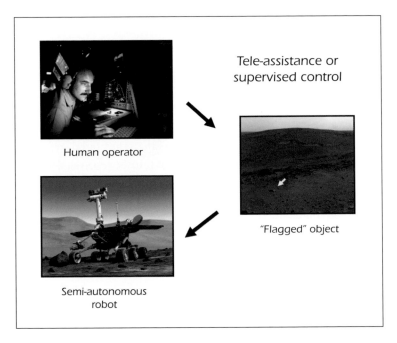

Figure 9.1 In tele-assistance, a human operator looks at a remote scene displayed on a video monitor. The video signal is provided by a camera mounted on a robot at the scene. If the operator notices an object of interest in the scene, she flags that object so that the robot can then locate it and retrieve it for later analysis. The operator needs to know little about the real distance and scale of the object; the robot can figure that out by itself using on-board optical sensors and range finders. By the same token, the robot needs to know nothing about the significance or meaning of the object it is retrieving. In our model of the visual system, the ventral stream and associated areas play a role analogous to that of the human operator, whereas the dorsal stream acts more like the robot.

operators can control robots working in hostile environments, such as in the crater of a volcano or on the surface of another planet. In tele-assistance, a human operator identifies and "flags" the goal object, such as an interesting rock on the surface of Mars, and then uses a symbolic language to communicate with a semi-autonomous robot that actually picks up the rock.

A robot working with tele-assistance is much more flexible than a completely autonomous robot. In some environments, of course, flexibility is not so important. Autonomous robots work well in situations such as an automobile assembly line, where the tasks they have to perform are highly constrained and well specified. These tasks can be quite complex and precise, depending on detailed sensory feedback from the actions performed. But autonomous robots can accomplish such highly precise operations only in the working environment for which they have been designed. They could not cope with events that its programmers had not anticipated. Imagine the difficulty, for example, of programming an autonomous robot so that it could deal with everything it might encounter on the surface of Mars. Clearly there is no way of anticipating all the possible objects and variations in terrain that it might confront. As a consequence, it might fail to react appropriately to critically important objects or events that it encounters. It would be oblivious to things that the scientists were not looking for in the first place, yet which might have been of great importance to investigate.

At present, the only way to make sure that the robot does the right thing in unforeseen circumstances is to have a human operator somewhere in the loop. One way to do this is to have the movements or instructions of the human operator (the master) simply reproduced in a one-to-one fashion by the robot (the slave). For instance, an operator in a nuclear plant might move a joystick that directly controls the movements of a robot arm in a radioactive laboratory. But such tele-operation, as this method of control is sometimes called, cannot cope well with sudden changes in scale (on the video monitor) or with a significant delay between the communicated action and feedback from that action. This is where tele-assistance comes into its own.

In tele-assistance the human operator doesn't have to worry about the real metrics of the workspace or the timing of the movements made by the robot; instead, the human operator has the job of identifying a goal and specifying an action toward that goal in general terms. Once this information is communicated to the semi-autonomous robot, the robot can use its on-board range finders and other sensing devices to work out the required movements for achieving the specified goal. In short, tele-assistance combines the flexibility of tele-operation with the precision of autonomous robotic control.

Our current conception of how the two visual streams interact in the animal or human brain is nicely analogous to this engineering principle. The perceptual systems

175

in the ventral stream, along with their associated memory and other higher-level cognitive systems in the brain, do a job rather like that of the human operator in tele-assistance. They identify different objects in the scene, using a representational system that is rich and detailed but not metrically precise. When a particular goal object has been flagged, dedicated visuomotor networks in the dorsal stream, in conjunction with output systems elsewhere in the brain (located in other brain structures including the premotor cortex, basal ganglia, and brainstem) are activated to perform the desired motor act. In other words, dorsal stream networks, with their precise egocentric coding of the location, size, orientation, and shape of the goal object, are like the robotic component of tele-assistance. Both systems have to work together in the production of purposive behavior—one system to help select the goal object from the visual array, the other to carry out the required metrical computations for the goal-directed action.

Of course in drawing this analogy with tele-assistance, we do not wish to underestimate the future possible developments in the design of autonomous robots. Clearly engineers are making great strides on this front. One day it is quite likely that the role of the human operator could be incorporated into the design of the machine. But how would you set about building such a super-robot? What kind of visual system should it have? The lessons learned from biology tell us that there would be little prospect of success in trying to give such a robot a general-purpose visual system, one that both recognizes objects in the world and guides the robot's movements. As we have argued throughout the book, the computational demands of object recognition and scene analysis are simply incompatible with the computational demands of visuomotor control. A much more effective design for the super-robot's visual system would be to emulate the division of labor between the ventral and dorsal visual streams in the primate brain.

There would need to be an intelligent processing module in the robot, one that can analyze scenes and select appropriate goals on the basis of both current input and information stored in its knowledge base (both built-in and learned). The most efficient way for this module to operate would be to construct a representation of the world based on relational metrics computed within a contextual or world-based frame of reference. But these computations, while crucially important for determining goals, would not be directly helpful in guiding the robot's actual movements in achieving those goals. To do this would require a separate set of dedicated and metrically precise sensorimotor modules, ones that are specialized for carrying out the just-in-time computations that determine the parameters of the specific actions required to achieve the specified goal. Only when such a super-robot is designed and built would the human operator become redundant. Then the robot could be truly said to be putting its thoughts into action.

176

In robotic tele-assistance, the human operator can communicate with the semi-autonomous robot via radio. The operator can flag the intended target by indicating its position on the video monitor at the control center. That position is not the location of the target in the real world of Mars but rather simply its position on the screen, which corresponds precisely to the robot's eye-view. The robot now has all the information it needs to zero-in on the object. The operator can then select the appropriate motor command from the robot's repertoire, such as "retrieve," and the robot does the rest. But what happens in a biological tele-assistance system like that found in the human brain? How does the ventral stream tell the dorsal stream what the target is and what to do with it?

Certainly there is good evidence from brain anatomy that the two streams are interconnected, through several direct and indirect routes. But just how the ventral stream flags the location of the intended target in a coordinate system that the dorsal stream can understand is not immediately obvious. After all, as we discussed in Chapter 8, the ventral stream works in scene-based coordinates and is more attuned to where an object is relative to other things in the world than where it is relative to the observer. But to control actions such as grasping, the dorsal stream has to know where an object is, not with respect to other objects, but rather with respect to the current position of the hand. And if it is going to control another kind of action such as kicking a ball, it has to know where the ball is with respect to the foot. So the two systems are using entirely different frames of reference—speaking a different language in fact—and yet somehow the ventral stream has to tell the dorsal stream which object to act upon.

One way that this could happen is by taking advantage of the fact that the information feeding into both systems comes from the same source—the retina and early visual areas such as primary visual cortex. These low-level visual processors contain a two-dimensional "snapshot" of whatever the eyes are looking at. Although this information is passed on separately to the two streams where it is used for different purposes, the pathways are actually two-way streets. In other words, there are lots of back-projections from higher-order areas in both streams back down to primary visual cortex. In fact it is now well established that the back-projections frequently outnumber the forward-going ones. This means that the two streams could communicate indirectly with one another via these back-projections to the shared origins of their incoming signals. Since these early signals are still coded in retinotopic coordinates, it would be possible for the ventral stream to flag a target for the dorsal stream using this common frame of reference. Once a target has been highlighted on the retinal map, it can be converted into any other coordinate system that the dorsal stream might need to use.

Imagine that a target for a grasping movement had been highlighted by the ventral stream in this way. Since the dorsal stream now knows where the target is on the retinal map, it can compute its location with respect to the hand. It might then go something like this. First the dorsal stream computes the position of eye with respect to the head, then the position of the head with respect to the body, and finally the position of the hand with respect to the body. It can now work out where the target is with respect to the hand. Similar kinds of computations could be used to compute where a soccer ball is located with respect to the foot. In other words, once the dorsal stream gets a fix on the retinal location of a goal object, it can transform that information in whatever way it needs to control a huge range of different actions. Although the dorsal and ventral streams have their own sophisticated and specialized languages, they both still retain contact with the more basic language of the retina. Rather like the human operator can instruct the robot via the two-dimensional optical array behind the lens of the robot's camera, so the ventral stream can instruct the dorsal stream via the common retinotopic map in early visual areas.

There is another likely player in this scenario—the lateral intraparietal area (LIP+)—the area in the dorsal stream that plays an important role in the visual control of eye movements (see Chapter 5, Figure 5.9). This area also seems to be critical for shifting our attention from one object to another in a visual scene, even when we don't move our eyes. In other words, the control of attention may have "piggy-backed"—in evolutionary terms—on the control of eye movements. Current functional magnetic resonance imaging (fMRI) evidence suggests that LIP+ somehow transmits the focus of its current attentional "searchlight" to the ventral stream, possibly again via downstream projections back to early visual areas, such as primary visual cortex. In fact, there is evidence from neurophysiological studies that when a monkey pays attention to a particular location, the activity of neurons corresponding to that location in primary visual cortex is enhanced. The way things look is that there is constant two-way traffic between the streams, and that an important route for this traffic is via the early visual areas with which both streams keep constantly in touch. Of course, it is also possible that area LIP+ would have the retinal coordinates by virtue of the fact that it has already got the attended target in its sights. Once higher-order brain areas (probably within the frontal lobes, which are known to play an important role in decision-making) give the command to act on the basis of visual information provided by the ventral stream, then the coordinate information in LIP+ could be accessed by the appropriate dorsal stream visuomotor areas for programming the action correctly.

All of this is highly speculative and over-simplified. We do not know for sure how the two streams communicate. But research on interactions between the two streams is well underway in visuomotor laboratories around the world, and holds the promise of explaining in detail how "seeing" and "doing" work together. The final answers to these questions will probably owe as much to detailed analyses of behavior as to neurobiological investigations.

Top-down control of action

In drawing this analogy with tele-assistance, we do not wish to imply that the ventral stream plays only a very remote role in the implementation of action, rather like a chief executive officer in a corporation, setting goals and writing mission statements and then delegating the real work to others. It does appear to keep the executive systems in the frontal lobes well informed in order to optimize the high-level planning of our actions, but the ventral stream itself also plays a hands-on role in many aspects of behavior.

The ventral stream contributes directly to certain aspects of motor programming, notably those that depend on information that cannot be derived in a bottom-up manner, directly from the retina. If you think about it for a moment, when you pick up an object, your fingers typically close around it with just enough force so that it will not slip out of your fingers when you lift it, but not so forcefully that you damage it. In other words, the force you apply has to be scaled appropriately for the object's weight (and its other characteristics) from the moment your fingers make contact, well before any feedback from touch and other somatosensory receptors comes into play. Unlike the size, location, orientation, or even shape of an object, which can be computed from the projected image on the retina, the object's mass, compliance (how hard or soft the object is), and surface friction can be gleaned only through experience. Take the case of two objects of roughly the same size but different weights: say a phone book and a box of crackers. You will automatically apply more grip force when you pick up the phone book than when you pick up the box of crackers. Of course, you already have a good idea about how heavy phone books and boxes of crackers are. But you can only make use of this knowledge to calibrate your grip force if you recognize the object in the first place. Such recognition, as we have seen, has to be carried out by visual mechanisms in the ventral, not the dorsal, stream.

But there is another twist to the story. When you pick up unfamiliar objects that are made of the same material but are not the same size, you typically apply more grip force to the larger object than you do to the smaller one—presumably because your brain makes the entirely reasonable assumption that the large object weighs more than the small one. At first sight, this might look like the kind of thing the dorsal stream could do on its own. After all, it already computes object size for scaling the opening of the hand in flight as it approaches the object. Why couldn't the dorsal stream simply use the information it already has about object size to scale grip force when you pick up the object? But this apparently straightforward task is beyond the visual capabilities of the dorsal stream, because more information than size is needed. The force you need to apply is determined not so much by the *size* of the object, as its weight. This means that the brain has to know about the properties of the material that the object is made of. Just like the phone book example, the brain has to use its stored visual knowledge about the density of different materials. For example, you would apply much greater force to pick up a rock than you would to pick up a piece of polystyrene of the same size (unless of course the polystyrene had been painted to look like a stone, as it might be on a film set—then you might get a surprise!).

So the brain's computation of the grip force required to pick up a particular object the first time is a joint product of visual size and stored knowledge about the density of the material from which that kind of object is typically made. The dorsal stream, which we know is dominated almost entirely by its current visual input, could never by itself compute the weight of an object. Of course, it is still possible that the dorsal stream computes the size of the object, even though it is the ventral stream that is needed to figure out what the object is made of. But it is equally possible that the ventral stream does both jobs. After all, it does compute size all the time in constructing our perceptual experience. So we are confronted with the question: Which stream computes size for grip force? One way to answer it is to see whether or not pictorial illusions, which are known to affect the perception of size but not the scaling of grip size, affect the scaling of grip force. If the dorsal stream controls the force as well as the size of the grip, then grip force should not be affected by the illusion. If the ventral stream provides the size information, however, then grip force, like perception, should be affected by the illusion.

Stephen Jackson, a psychologist at the University of Nottingham, UK, carried out this very experiment. To do this, he used the Ponzo illusion, in which an object placed within the converging end of the two lines looks larger than one placed within the diverging end (see Chapter 8, Figure 8.4). As expected, when people reached out to pick up an object placed in these two different positions, their grip aperture was scaled to the real, not the perceived size of the object. What surprised Jackson, however, was that their grip force *was* affected by the illusion. In other words, his subjects scaled their grip force to the perceived, not the real size of the object, applying more force when the object looked (deceptively) bigger. So the question about which visual stream computes grip force seems to have been answered—the whole job is done by the ventral stream. Consistent with this, we have found that Dee Fletcher has real problems with adjusting her grip force when objects of different size are used—that is, when she has only *visual* information about the size. When she can also *feel* the object's size, she adjusts her grip appropriately.

The semantics of action

When you pick up a knife, you usually pick it up by the handle, not the blade. When you pick up a screwdriver you do the same thing even though, unlike the knife, there is no danger of cutting yourself. In other words, many objects, especially tools, elicit (or "afford," to use a term coined by the perceptual psychologist James J. Gibson) "use-appropriate" actions. Even when the screwdriver is positioned with its handle pointing away from you, you will typically turn your hand right around in a slightly awkward fashion and grasp it by the handle as if you were about to use it (see Figure 9.2). It goes further than that. Your intentions come into the equation as well. Say you are going to put the knife into your dishwasher. If you intend to make sure that the blade of the knife is pointing upwards in the rack, then you will probably grab it by the blade (carefully) when you take it off the table. In short, the function of an object and what you intend to do with it will dictate how you pick it up.

But when you are faced with an object, how does the brain know what the appropriate way to grasp it is? First and foremost, the brain has to know what the object

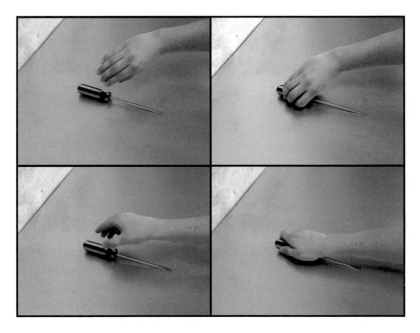

Figure 9.2 When we pick up a screwdriver, we typically grab it by the handle, even when it is pointed away from us. In the picture on the upper left, the person picks up the screwdriver with a hand posture that is awkward but is well suited to the use to which the screwdriver will be put (upper right). When the person is preoccupied with a memory task, however, he or she will often pick up the screwdriver using a well-formed grasp but one that is unrelated to tool use.

is. This is clearly a job for the ventral stream. But an important part of recognizing what an object is, particularly a manufactured object, is knowing what it is *for* (that is, its "functional semantics"). This means there must be links between the ventral stream and our stored information about how the hand should grip the object in order to use it. The use of these functional semantics in selecting the appropriate grasp has been shown in an elegant experiment carried out by Sarah Creem and Dennis Proffitt at the University of Virginia, USA. They presented undergraduate volunteers with a series of tools and implements, such as a toothbrush, a frying pan, and a screwdriver, with the handles turned away from them. Needless to say, when the students reached out to pick up these objects, they still grabbed the handle even though this meant adopting an uncomfortable posture. If, however, they were doing this while they simultaneously tried to recall words they had learned before, they picked up the object as if blind to its functional semantics. Nonetheless, although they grasped the objects inappropriately, they still picked them up deftly, showing well-calibrated grasps. In other words, the dorsal stream was still doing its job as well as ever—it was just the functional aspects that were missing. They were missing presumably because the word-memory task was putting heavy demands on the high-level cognitive processes needed to retrieve the functional semantics of the object and thus the appropriate grasp to use. Indeed, Creem and Proffitt showed in another experiment that tasks which did not have a large semantic component but which nevertheless demanded the students' attention did not interfere with the functional aspects of their grasps.

These results strongly suggest that it is the ventral rather than the dorsal stream that provides us with visual information about the function of an object. If this is so, then we would expect that someone whose ventral stream is damaged, such as Dee Fletcher, would pick up functional objects rather like the students did in Creem and Proffitt's experiment when they were engrossed in the word-memory task. In other words, she should make "grasp mistakes" when asked to pick up manufactured objects such as a knife or a screwdriver that are oriented with the handle pointing away. In fact, Dee does show mistakes of this kind. When she reaches out to pick up such objects (ones she cannot identify by sight), her grasp is perfectly matched to the object's size, shape, and orientation, but shows no indication that she understands its function. Thus, she grasps the screwdriver by its shaft rather than its handle— and only then rotates it in her hand so that she can hold it properly. In other words, because her damaged ventral stream is unable to process the screwdriver's shape, Dee has no idea what it is ahead of time and is therefore unable to generate an appropriate grasping movement. Nevertheless, the intact visuomotor systems in her dorsal stream can still compute the required metrics to ensure that her grasping movement, however inappropriate, is well formed and efficient.

We mentioned earlier that when the ventral stream has identified an object for the dorsal stream to act upon, the two streams probably share information about the object's location through early cortical areas like V1, which both streams are connected to, or via LIP+. But we have just seen in this section that the ventral stream also needs to send signals to the dorsal stream of a higher order, about *what kind of object* is being selected. In other words it needs to communicate not only *where* the object is but also *what* the object is (and what to do with it). This probably requires other kinds of connections between the two streams, via circuits that include higher-cognitive areas in the prefrontal cortex. We have known from anatomical studies since the 1970s that strong connections between these brain regions do exist. These links, involving higher-order cognitive areas, could guide the dorsal stream, for example, in its selection of the appropriate way to pick the object up. It is interesting to note that recent fMRI studies show that brain areas in both the ventral and the dorsal streams are activated equally by pictures of tools and by appropriate tool-directed actions. But in the end, it is the ventral, not the dorsal, stream that must provide the perceptual information for selecting the appropriate action to make when confronted with a functional object such as a tool.

So is the ventral stream a visuomotor system as well?

Well no, not exactly. But ultimately everything the brain does is done in the service of action. Otherwise brains would never have evolved at all. As we pointed out in Chapter 4, natural selection operates on the consequences of action, not on the consequences of thought alone. The ventral stream makes contributions to action in several ways. For example, it is the ventral stream that identifies the goal objects for action, and that enables the brain to select the class of action to perform. The ventral stream, as we have seen, also plays the dominant role in deciding how much force to apply when picking things up, and probably also how hard we kick a soccer ball.

In practice it is going to be very difficult to tease apart the different elements that are contributed by the two streams even in an apparently simple everyday action like picking up a coffee cup. For example, it is your ventral stream that allows you to identify the objects on the table and to distinguish your cup from others that might be there. It is your ventral stream, too, that allows you to single out the handle from the rest of the cup, so that you can then select the appropriate hand posture for picking up the cup to take a drink of coffee. But having identified the handle of your cup and the action you wish to perform, it is then up to the visuomotor machinery in the dorsal stream to get your hand and fingers positioned efficiently on the cup's handle. In addition to this, the scaling of the initial forces that you apply to lift the cup to your mouth is based on the stored information about the weight of the cup, which you have to access through your ventral stream. So although your dorsal stream takes the responsibility for transforming the visual metrics of the goal into a smooth and efficient movement, your ventral stream does not remain aloof and uninvolved. It is closely involved in our actions at all levels, not just at the planning stage but right down to the programming of the force we apply with our fingers.

Conscious and unconscious vision

We began the book by introducing Dee Fletcher, a young woman who has lost all visual experience of the shapes of objects. We have often asked Dee what the world looks like to her. She finds it very hard to put it into words. As we mentioned earlier, she sometimes says that things "run into each other" so that she finds it hard to tell where one object ends and the other begins, especially when the two objects have a similar color or are made from the same material. She also mentions that things often look "fuzzy" to her. But, as we noted, it is not like the experience that a short-sighted person has when he takes off his glasses. Do not forget that Dee has excellent acuity—she can see fine detail. The problem may be that we are asking Dee to talk about what she doesn't see—we are asking her to describe what is *not* there in her conscious experience. The same questions have been asked of patients with blindsight. These people have a complete absence of visual experience in the visual field opposite their brain damage. But they do not say that everything on that side looks blank or that there's some kind of hole in their field of vision. They find the question impossible to answer. Just as you would find it impossible to say what you "see" beyond the edges of your visual field, or behind your back. So perhaps we are expecting too much of Dee when we ask her what she sees. She cannot describe what she cannot see.

Yet despite the fact that Dee has no conscious visual experience of object shape, she retains the ability to use information about the shape to guide her actions. Dee's case, along with evidence from a broad range of studies from frogs to humans, tells us that visual perception and the visual control of action depend on quite different brain systems. What we have learned from these studies is that conscious visual experience of the world is a product of the ventral not the dorsal stream. You might perceive the tennis ball that has just been lobbed over the net by your opponent, but you can never be conscious of the specific information that your visuomotor system uses to guide your successful return. This visuomotor computation happens entirely unconsciously. You are not aware of the fact that the ball is expanding at a certain rate on your retina and that this is an important cue for knowing exactly when to swing to hit it with the "sweet spot" of the racquet. When you are running around the court chasing the ball, the visual scene is changing on your retina quite dramatically. The shape of the projected image of the net, for example, will be constantly changing—and yet you will continue to see the net as a stable and unchanging object in the scene. It is perhaps a good thing that you are *not* aware of all of these viewer-dependent changes. If you were, the world would become a bewildering kaleidoscope of unrelated and disconnected experiences in which objects change their sizes and shapes as you move about. What you need are the enduring constancies of perception in order to make sense of the world.

But how does the ventral stream give us that elusive mental quality of "awareness"? This raises the general question: How can physical states in *any* part of the brain give rise to conscious states? These questions present philosophical and empirical problems that are currently impossible to solve. Nonetheless, the first experimental steps in approaching these questions have already been taken. These first steps skirt around the philosophical minefields by only asking what *correlations* may exist between brain states and mental states. The hoary question of how one causes the other is shelved for future investigators to grapple with. Admittedly, even this correlational question still has a long way to go before being answered convincingly. Scientists are addressing it by building on the most solid knowledge we have about the brain. This means that the question has to be focused on particular kinds of mental processes. A broad approach, aimed at explaining conscious states in general, is just too ambitious at present. Although that broader question remains one of the ultimate aims of brain research, it will have to await a general account of brain function. Such an account, a kind of "theory of everything" for neurobiology, is a goal that science has not yet even begun to approach.

This brings us back to the visual system, which at the present time is undoubtedly the best-understood system in the brain. As we have tried to show in this book, the past 30 years has seen enormous breakthroughs in our knowledge of the neuroscience of visual processing. So much so that research on the brain's visual system probably offers us the best way forward for attacking the problem of consciousness. This approach was famously advocated by the Nobel laureate Francis Crick and the neurobiologist Christof Koch during the 1990s. Crick and Koch encapsulated the problem by posing the questions "What is it about the brain systems mediating visual processing that makes their activity conscious?" and "What is it about the brain activity underlying visual processing that makes it conscious under some conditions but unconscious under others?"

Of course, much of the work on the details of the visual brain has come from work in animals, particularly monkeys. In fact the wiring diagram of the ventral stream was initially worked out in the monkey. But tracing pathways in the monkey brain is one thing, determining what the monkey experiences is quite another. Humans can describe what they experience, monkeys cannot. So how do we show that in monkeys, just as in humans, the ventral stream plays the key role in constructing their visual experience? It is certainly difficult, but it's not impossible.

Finding correlations between brain activity and consciousness

There is an ingenious example of how it can be done. It provides direct evidence that what a monkey reports seeing is directly related to neuronal activity in the highest regions of the ventral stream. As we saw in Chapter 4, neurons in the inferior temporal cortex of the monkey respond selectively to images like faces, colored shapes, and different kinds of objects. Nikos Logothetis and his colleagues in Germany have shown that the activity of these neurons is closely linked to the perceptual experience of the monkey. They first trained the monkey to report, by pressing a lever, which of two alternative images it saw on a screen in front of it, over a period of 30 minutes or so. Sometimes one image would appear, say a picture of a face, sometimes the other, say a sunburst pattern; and whenever the picture changed, the monkey had to press the appropriate lever. Once the monkeys had learned this, the experimenters presented both images simultaneously, one to each eye, causing "binocular rivalry" (see Figure 9.3). When different incompatible images like this are simultaneously presented to the two eyes, a person hardly ever sees a fused combination of the two, but instead sees either the complete face or the complete sunburst pattern. It is as if the two pictures are competing with each other for consciousness. Sometime you are conscious of one, sometimes the other: the two percepts alternate with each other at intervals of a few seconds or so. When Logothetis's experimental animal was faced with this binocular rivalry, it alternately reported seeing one of the two images, then the other, just as a human would.

The exciting discovery was that the responses of inferior temporal neurons followed the monkey's perceptual reports with a high correlation. Even though the images never changed physically on the screen, the monkey's reports of what it saw changed repeatedly—and these changes correlated with fluctuations in the activity of neurons deep in the ventral stream, specifically in the inferior temporal cortex. For example, a neuron that preferred faces responded strongly when the monkey reported seeing the face and weakly when it reported seeing the sunburst, and vice versa. But neurons earlier in the system, like area V1, did not show these correlations. At that level neurons responded in the same way no matter what the monkey indicated that it saw. Even in intermediate areas such as V4, early in the ventral stream, the correlations were relatively weak.

It remains true of course that whereas details of the brain are more easily studied in animals, the niceties of consciousness are more easily studied in humans. Yet

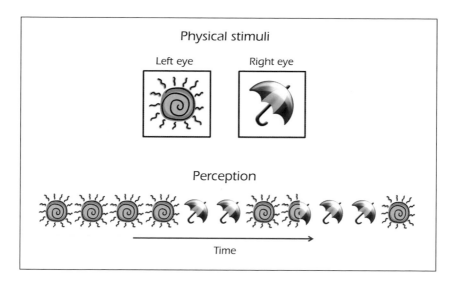

Figure 9.3 When incompatible images (top) are shown separately to our two eyes, we tend to alternate between seeing one and seeing the other (bottom). Rarely, but occasionally, do we see a composite of two images. This alternation between incompatible percepts is called "binocular rivalry" and has proved useful for studying the neural correlates of visual consciousness.

whenever comparisons are made between the activity in visual areas in the monkey and the human, we see very similar things happening. This is perhaps unsurprising given the extent of our evolutionary heritage that humans share with monkeys. Nonetheless, it is important that findings like those of Logothetis be followed up in humans to see if the activity in our ventral stream also reflects our conscious visual experience. For obvious reasons it is difficult to look at the activity of single neurons in the human brain. But the advent of brain imaging techniques like fMRI makes it possible to measure the activity of large groups of neurons that share common visual properties. For example, as we saw in Chapter 5, Nancy Kanwisher and her colleagues used fMRI to delineate two ventral-stream areas, one called the fusiform face area (FFA), which is selectively activated by pictures of faces, and another area, the parahippocampal place area (PPA), which is activated mostly by pictures of houses or scenes. She used this difference between the two areas to study the changes in visual consciousness during binocular rivalry in much the same way as Logothetis had done in the monkey. Kanwisher, together with her colleague Frank Tong and others, scanned the brains of volunteers while showing them pictures of a face and a house simultaneously, one picture to each eye (see Figure 9.4). Just like Logothetis's monkeys, sometimes the volunteers would see the house and sometimes

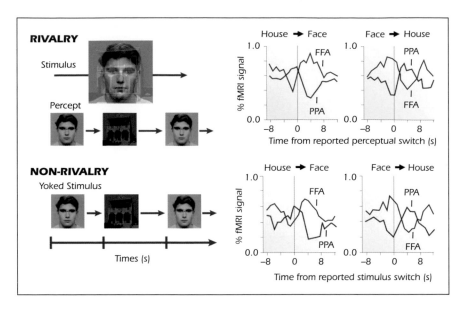

Figure 9.4 This figure shows the results of an fMRI study using binocular rivalry (see Figure 9.3). Brain activation was measured in the FFA (selective for faces) and the PPA (selective for buildings) when observers viewed rivalrous images of a face and of a house (top left). The level of activation switched between the two brain areas in step with what the observers reported seeing (top right). The changes in activation in the two areas were just the same as those seen when the two pictures were presented successively (rather than simultaneously) in a manner mimicking the alternations of rivalry (bottom left and right). Reprinted from *Neuron*, 21(4), Frank Tong, Ken Nakayama, J. Thomas Vaughan, and Nancy Kanwisher, Binocular rivalry and visual awareness in human extrastriate cortex, pp. 753–759, Figure 1. © (1998), with permission from Elsevier.

the face, but almost never both at once. They were asked to press a key whenever one percept was replaced by the other. Whenever the volunteers reported seeing the face, there was more activity in their FFA—but when they reported seeing the house, there was more activity in their PPA. In other words, the activity in the FFA and the PPA reflected what they consciously perceived, not what was on their retina (which never changed).

Tim Andrews, then at the University of Durham, UK, addressed the same kind of question, but using the ambiguous "face/vase" figure shown in Figure 9.5. Just like our perception of the competing images in binocular rivalry, our perception of this ambiguous figure changes from moment to moment. Sometimes we see a vase on a dark background and sometimes we see two profile faces against a light background. But we never see both at once. Andrews took advantage of the fact that objects like the vase activate a different area in the human ventral stream, the lateral

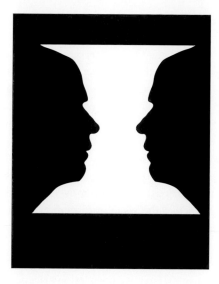

Figure 9.5 The famous face/vase picture, devised by Edgar Rubin, a Danish psychologist, is an example of an ambiguous figure. Sometimes we see two black faces against a white background, and sometimes we see a white vase against a black background. We cannot see both at once. This ambiguous figure, like binocular rivalry displays, has been used to study the neural basis of visual consciousness.

occipital area (LO: see Chapter 5). He presented volunteers with the face/vase figure to look at for a few minutes, asking them to press a key every time they saw the faces change to a vase or vice versa, and contrasted the activity in area LO with activity in the FFA. The results were clear. The changes in perception were closely correlated with activity changes between the FFA and area LO. In other words, although these observers were looking at an unchanging screen, their brain activity kept switching between the FFA and area LO. And when this happened, what the observers consciously saw changed as well.

Of course, none of this fMRI research demonstrates that *only* the ventral stream is associated with conscious visual processing, since the dorsal stream wasn't usually tested. Yet pictures of objects can activate areas in the dorsal stream too—including area hAIP, where visual information about objects drives the formation of our grasping movements (see Chapter 5). Recently, Fang Fang and Sheng He at the University of Minnesota have asked the question whether levels of activation in these dorsal stream areas are correlated with awareness or unawareness just as activations in the ventral stream are. In their study, instead of pitting two different patterns against each other, one shown to the left eye and the other to the right, Fang and He created "interocular suppression" by presenting high-contrast dynamic noise to just one eye. This noise (rather like the appearance of a TV screen when no signal is getting through from a TV station) prevented the observers from consciously seeing pictures of objects that were presented to the other eye. Yet these pictures still elicited substantial fMRI activation in the dorsal stream—and more importantly this activation was just as great as when there was no interocular suppression (i.e. the pictures were consciously perceived). It is important to note that, as we would expect from previous work, Fang and He did find large differences in activation in the ventral stream area LO between these "aware" and "unaware" testing conditions. So it seems that the dorsal stream responds to visual objects indistinguishably in both the "conscious" and "unconscious" test conditions. Its activations remain the same, quite independently of whether the visual information is perceived consciously or not. That distinction seems to be entirely the ventral stream's business.

In summary, we have converging evidence from three kinds of research that allows us to be rather confident that neural activity in the ventral stream is closely correlated with visual consciousness. First, we have lesion evidence: this shows us that the ventral stream is a necessary part of the circuitry for visual awareness. Without the ventral stream, there is no visual consciousness. Second, we know from fMRI evidence that fluctuations in visual awareness are closely correlated with changes in the activation of different areas within the ventral stream. And third, we have evidence from single-neuron recordings in monkeys that the activity of cells in inferotemporal cortex is tightly linked to perceptual fluctuations. While this latter evidence is indirect in that we can only assume that the monkey's visual experience resembles our own, nonetheless studies of this kind provide our first real handle on what may be happening at the level of individual neurons. Together, these three lines of inquiry give us a convincing lead on *where* in the brain neuronal activity correlates with visual awareness. But of course they do not explain what it is about the neurons in the ventral stream that gives them this property.

After all, none of these studies shows that ventral stream activation is *always* associated with awareness. On the contrary, they show quite the opposite. Consider the fate of a picture that has lost out at a given moment in the competition between left and right eyes during binocular rivalry. Not only does this suppressed picture still activate early areas of the visual cortex like V1, it also still activates to some extent the relevant ventral-stream areas (FFA for faces, PPA for places, or area LO for objects). In other words, the activation goes up or down according to whether the stimulus is conscious or unconscious, but it never actually disappears completely. So why is ventral-stream activity sometimes conscious and sometimes unconscious? It could, of course, be that the sheer *amount* of activity in a particular ventral-stream area determines whether or not its activity leads to a conscious experience. Alternatively, it could be that the activity in that area has to be synchronized with activity elsewhere in the brain, either earlier visual areas like V1, and/or higher-order structures such as the frontal lobes. There is a lot of speculation about such possibilities, but to date there is a shortage of convincing empirical evidence to support any particular hypothesis.

So we have no real idea what the critical difference is between neural activity that reaches awareness and that which does not. But certainly visual information that does not reach awareness does get processed to quite a high level of analysis in the ventral stream. This processing could well account for so-called unconscious perception, in which subliminal (subjectively unseen) stimuli can influence behavior. For example, seeing a subliminal image of a cat speeds up your reaction to a semantically related image like a dog, when you are being asked to classify pictures as animate or inanimate, by making a quick key-press. This means that your brain has in some sense *seen* the cat well enough to activate your semantic database about animals. But what should be emphasized here is that although unconscious perception does seem to occur, it arises from activity within the ventral, not the dorsal stream. In fact, the visual computations underlying unconscious perception seem to be identical to those underlying conscious perception: it's just that they do not make it into awareness.

So what about visually elicited activity in the dorsal stream? We have seen that this activity does not give rise to visual awareness, but that doesn't mean that it could give rise to unconscious perception. Use of that phrase carries an implication that the visual processing could *in principle* be conscious. The fact is that visual activity in the dorsal stream can never become conscious—so "perception" is just the wrong word to use. The dorsal stream is not in the business of providing any kind of a visual representation of the world—it just converts visual information directly into action. The visual processing that it carries out is no more accessible to conscious scrutiny than the visual processing that elicits the pupillary light reflex. Dorsal-stream processing is more complex than that which supports the pupillary light reflex, but in the end they are both simply visuomotor control systems with no more pretensions to consciousness than we see in the robot in a tele-assistance network. It is the human operator (the ventral stream with linked cognitive systems) that provides the conscious monitoring of what's going on, even though it is the robot (the dorsal stream) that is doing the work.

Is the visual processing that guides our actions truly unconscious?

The idea that we can see our coffee cup clearly and consciously, yet at the same time not be using that same visual percept to guide our act of picking it up, is highly counter-intuitive. After all, it seems perfectly obvious that our visual experience of the coffee cup and the visual information that controls our grasp are one and the same. The British philosopher, Andy Clark, has called this mistaken idea the "assumption of experience-based control." Nevertheless, many people, even some eminent visual scientists, steadfastly refuse to abandon this assumption. And of course it is very difficult to demonstrate the fallacy here, since our perceptions are normally so tightly correlated with our visual behavior. It is only when the two are split apart artificially, as we saw in Chapter 8 in visual illusions, that we can begin to get close to demonstrating in the dissociation between perception and action in healthy people.

Of course, such dissociations, as we have seen, are shown most clearly in individuals with damage to either the dorsal or the ventral stream. But another way of probing the question is to test brain-damaged people who have a visual symptom known as "extinction." One such patient was Victor Edelman, an elderly man who had suffered a right-hemisphere stroke a year before we tested him. Immediately after the stroke, Victor showed several signs of visual neglect (see Chapter 3, Box 3.1), often failing to notice objects presented in the left side of space. This neglect recovered completely, however, and Victor's only residual symptom when we met him was sensory extinction. This meant that whenever we showed him two flashes of light, for example, one on the left and one on the right, he would often say that he didn't see the one on the left. Yet when only one light was flashed, on either side, he reported it almost every time. Extinction is thought to be a kind of imbalance of attention, such that when there is competition between two different events, it is the one on the side of visual space opposite the brain damage that loses out and doesn't make it into consciousness. The fact that an event on the "bad" side can be perceived when it is presented by itself shows that there is no visual field deficit per se, as is seen in patients with damage to the primary visual cortex V1. And indeed in Victor's case, careful testing with a perimeter (see Chapter 6) showed that there were no "blind" areas anywhere in his visual field.

For our first study of Victor, our colleague Rob McIntosh devised a new version of his obstacle avoidance board in which subjects were asked to reach between two potential obstacles to touch a gray strip at the back of the board (see Chapter 3.) But in this case we wanted to make the obstacles less easily seen, so that Victor would sometimes fail to detect the one on the left. So instead of thick cylinders, we used thin metal rods—and instead of giving enough time to see them clearly, we let Victor glimpse them for only a brief half-second (see Figure 9.6). Under these conditions Victor often failed to see the rod on the left—but not on every occasion. This meant we could compare the reaching movements he made when he saw both rods with those that he made when he saw only the one on the right. Also, on some occasions, only one rod was actually present, either on the left or the right. Just like a healthy

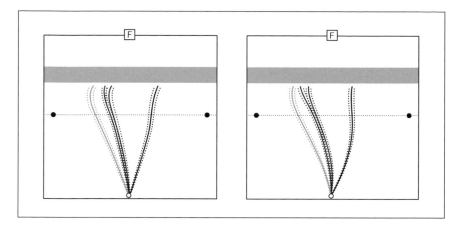

Figure 9.6 The movements made by our extinction patient Victor, when reaching between two thin rods to touch a gray strip at the back of the testing board. As can be seen, Victor steered a similar middle course when both rods were present, whether he consciously saw the one on the left (the trajectory shown in blue) or not (the trajectory shown in red). On those reaches, shown in red, when he didn't detect the left rod due to extinction, his reaches were well to the right of those made when there really *was* no left rod there (shown in green). (The trajectory shown in black depicts his reaches on trials when only the left rod was present.) From McIntosh, R.D., McClements, K.I., Schindler, I., Cassidy, T.P., Birchall, D., and Milner, A.D. (2004). Avoidance of obstacles in the absence of visual awareness. *Proceedings of the Royal Society, 271*, 15–20, Figure 2.

person, Victor moved his hand along quite different routes depending on whether the left, right, or both rods were present. Amazingly, when both rods were present, Victor's hand took exactly the same route, whether he consciously saw the left rod or not. Equally importantly, the routes his hand followed on trials on which he failed to perceive the rod on the left were quite different from those on which there really was no rod on the left (i.e. only one on the right). Evidently although Victor didn't see the left rod on many trials in which both rods were actually present, his visuomotor system did.

The second study, this one carried out by Thomas Schenk, asked about a quite different aspect of visually guided reaching—not whether an environmental object needed to be consciously seen for it to be taken into account, but instead whether the reaching hand itself needed to be consciously seen. It has been known for many years that when reaching out to a small target, people are more accurate when they can see their own hand during the reach than when they can't. The question we asked was whether this online visual feedback from the hand needed to be conscious in order for the improved accuracy to occur. Schenk devised a cunning way to exploit Victor's extinction so that he wouldn't always "see" his reaching hand.

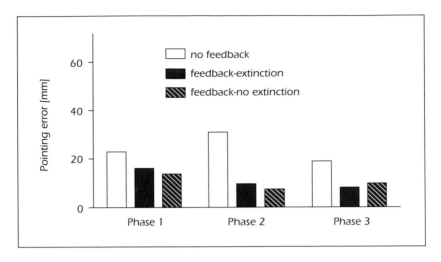

Figure 9.7 The average errors made by Victor when pointing to an LED target in the dark, while another LED was attached to his pointing finger. When the finger LED was switched on during the reach (solid and hatched bars), errors were reliably smaller than when it wasn't on (white bars). This means that Victor reached more accurately when he could visually monitor his hand during reaching. Importantly, this same benefit of visual feedback was there no matter whether Victor consciously saw the hand LED (hatched bars) or not (solid bars). This result held true for all three phases of the experiment where the experimental conditions were varied slightly in the dark. Reprinted from *Brain Research*, 1067(1), Ayten Türkkani Tunç, Mehmet Turgut, Hüseyin Aslan, Bünyamin Sahin, Mine Ertem Yurtseven, and Süleyman Kaplan, Neonatal pinealectomy induces Purkinje cell loss in the cerebellum of the chick: a stereological study, pp. 95–102, Figure 3. © (2006), with permission from Elsevier.

He had Victor reach in the dark toward an LED target with his left hand, and on half of the reaches a second LED attached to the forefinger of that hand was switched on during the reach (see Figure 9.7). On these occasions, there would be competition between the two LEDs for Victor's attention, and because of his extinction problem, he would often, but not always, fail to perceive the one on his hand.

First we confirmed that Victor's accuracy really did improve when the finger LED was on. It did—in fact the average size of Victor's reaching errors was about half of what they were when the finger LED was off, just like healthy subjects. So was there any difference between his reaches on trials where he perceived the LED on his hand and those where he didn't? It turned out that it didn't make any difference at all: he was just as accurate on trials when he consciously saw the hand LED as he was on trials when he didn't.

Both of these two studies with Victor followed a similar logic, in that we were able to compare occasions when Victor was or was not able to consciously see an important aspect of visual input when performing reaches toward a target. And the results were the same in both cases, demonstrating that the visual information was processed equally efficiently for the control of action whether he consciously perceived it or not. The conclusion seems inescapable: the visuomotor system in our dorsal stream guides our everyday movements with visual information that is not accessible to consciousness. It just gets on with the job. Our conscious experience is simply irrelevant.

Summary

We have tried in this book to make a strong case for the idea that vision is not unitary, and that our visual phenomenology reflects only one aspect of what the visual brain is doing. Much of what vision does for us lies outside our visual experience. Indeed, most of our actions are controlled by essentially robotic systems that use visual computations that are completely inaccessible to conscious scrutiny. This might sound at first glance rather like Cartesian dualism—the existence of a conscious mind separate from a reflexive machine. But the separation we are suggesting has nothing to do with the mind/brain distinction that Descartes espoused. Although the two kinds of visual processing are separate, both are embodied in the hardware of the brain.

The emphasis in much of the work we have described in this book has been on the differences between the two visual streams in the cerebral cortex—establishing where they go, why they are there, and how they work. This side of the story has depended crucially on evidence from patients like Dee who have suffered damage to one or the other stream. However, as we have tried to show in this chapter, there are complex but seamless interactions between the ventral perception stream and the dorsal action stream in the production of adaptive behavior. In the future, the most exciting advances are likely to come from applying new investigative methods to the task of learning how these interactions take place in providing us with a unified visual life.

Further Reading

Feedback as well as feedforward neural connections are likely to play a crucial role in the integration of activity in the two visual streams. For a recent account of the possible role of feedback connections in visual processing, see:

Lamme, V.A.F. (2006). Towards a true neural stance on consciousness. *Trends in Cognitive Sciences, 10,* 494–501.

This article by Michael Goldberg and colleagues shows how areas in the dorsal stream that are closely linked to the control of eye movements also play an important role in the shifting of attention from one object to another:

Goldberg, M.E., Bisley, J.W., Powell, K.D., and Gottlieb, J. (2006). Saccades, salience and attention: the role of the lateral intraparietal area in visual behavior. *Progress in Brain Research*, *155*, 157–175.

In this paper, the authors review evidence showing how perceptual information from the ventral stream is integrated with information processed by the dorsal stream in the production of skilled motor acts:

Goodale, M.A. and Haffenden, A.M. (2003). Interactions between the dorsal and ventral streams of visual processing. *Advances in Neurology*, *93*, 249–267.

The late Nobel laureate Francis Crick devoted the latter part of his scientific career to pursuing the neural basis of consciousness. A flavor of his approach to the problem can be gleaned from the following article that he wrote with his long-time collaborator Christof Koch:

Crick, F. and Koch, C. (2003). A framework for consciousness. *Nature Neuroscience*, *6*, 119–126.

Christof Koch has also written a highly accessible book that discusses these ideas:

Koch, C. (2003). *The Quest for Consciousness: A neurobiological approach.* Englewood, CO: Roberts and Company.

The following paper shows how empirical methods can be used to study the neural correlates of perceptual experience in the monkey. Using a combination of a clever behavioral training procedure along with single-neuron recording techniques, Nikos Logothetis was able to show that neural activity in high-level areas of the ventral stream is related directly to visual awareness:

Logothetis, N.K. (1998). Single units and conscious vision. *Philosophical Transactions of the Royal Society of London B: Biological Sciences*, *353*, 1801–1818.

Frank Tong, working in Nancy Kanwisher's lab, transferred this idea for relating brain activity to fluctuating perceptual experience to humans using fMRI in the following study:

Tong, F., Nakayama, K., Vaughan, J.T., and Kanwisher, N. (1998). Binocular rivalry and visual awareness in human extrastriate cortex. *Neuron*, *21*, 753–759.

The following book chapter provides a broad review and discussion of our own views on how the two visual streams contribute to our experience of visual consciousness:

Milner, A.D. (2008). Visual awareness and human action. In L. Weiskrantz and M. Davies (eds) *Frontiers in Consciousness Research*, pp. 169–214. Oxford: Oxford University Press.

(The book also contains several other chapters that will be of interest to any reader interested in exploring modern empirical and philosophical research on human consciousness.)

The following book discusses many of the same issues we have covered but also discusses some of the philosophical implications:

Jacob, P. and Jeannerod, M. (2003). *Ways of Seeing: The scope and Limits of visual cognition*. Oxford: Oxford University Press.

X

Postscript: Dee's life
Twenty-five years on

If you were a visitor at Dee's home today, you would find it hard to believe that she had any visual problems at all. She would welcome you at the door, invite you in, and no doubt show you around their now fully renovated house, including Carlo's wine cellar (converted from an original 17th-century structure), his pride and joy. She would almost certainly give you a guided tour of her garden—which is *her* pride and joy. She would walk you confidently down the path, pausing here and there to point out a particularly beautiful plant or flowering shrub. A little later, in the kitchen, as she made you a cup of tea, you would again see little sign of the devastating loss of form perception that we described earlier in this book. She would have no problem putting the kettle on the stove, finding the tea, milk, and sugar, and pouring the boiling water into the teapot. She would need no help in bringing the tray out to the terrace, where she would pour you a cup of tea. In fact, Dee in all these activities behaves so naturally and ably that you would never suspect that she had ever suffered the devastating loss of sight that she did. Of course she could always do much more than her conscious sight would seem to allow, even from early on. But her repertoire of visual skills has improved by leaps and bounds over the years since her accident. Her self-confidence and sureness of touch have increased steadily, hand in hand with these developing skills.

It is an important research question in itself to work out how it is that anyone who has suffered major brain damage can show such dramatic improvements over the years. Of course, some of the things that Dee can do are fairly easily explained. As we have seen in this book, Dee has a well-functioning visuomotor system. Using this system, she can still use vision to negotiate her way through a garden replete with paths and flowerbeds and to guide hand movements like picking up the kettle or handing you a teacup. But although this explains how she picks up the kettle, it doesn't explain how she selected the kettle in the first place. It also doesn't explain why she is so much better at everyday tasks now than she was twenty years ago, right after the accident.

One of the ways Dee can do this is not at all mysterious. Just like any person whose vision suddenly becomes impaired, she makes life easier for herself by making sure that things in the kitchen and around the rest of the house are kept in the same place from day to day. In conjunction with this commonsense strategy, she has the advantage over a blind person that she can guide her movements accurately to such objects without having to depend on memory and touch. She can do much more than this, however. For example, she can choose between two or more objects that happen to be on the counter—picking up the teacup instead of the coffee mug, for example. It helps a great deal that many things in the world have distinctive colors— and Dee still has vivid color perception. She has no trouble identifying flowers—and even foliage—by subtle differences in their color and visual texture. The same is true of many manufactured objects in the kitchen and tool shed, which again often have distinctive colors and sheens. It seems that although Dee is using a more limited repertoire of visual channels to help her identify objects, she does still see a world of objects—even if she sometimes makes mistakes and sees two adjacent objects as a single one. She does not just see an abstract melange or patchwork of different colors and textures.

But Dee has other ways of telling things apart that are not so obvious to the observer or even to her. We accidentally encountered an example of these more subtle strategies when testing her in the laboratory several years ago, using our usual "Efron blocks." In the particular experiment we were doing, she was asked to reach out and pick up a square block presented alongside a rectangular one of the same overall area (or vice versa). We didn't expect her to be able to do this. After all, she couldn't consciously distinguish between the two blocks. To our surprise, she reached out and picked up the right one much more often than she could have done by simply guessing. How did she know which one to pick up, when in other tests she couldn't tell us which was which? The secret was revealed when we noticed that she sometimes reached toward the wrong block but then corrected herself in midstream. When we examined videotapes of her movements, we discovered that this self-correction happened quite often—and when it did she was almost always correct on that particular occasion. In fact, when we examined only those occasions where she went straight for one of the blocks, her performance fell to chance. So what was going on here? We think she must have been somehow monitoring the posture of her hand as she reached out toward one of the blocks. If it didn't "feel" right she simply switched mid-flight to the other block. In other words, she was using feedback from her own finger movements to tell her whether the object she was heading for was the correct one. Having calibrated the action using her visuomotor system, which was able to compute the width of the object, she could use feedback from her action to help her make the correct choice. Dee wasn't deliberately cheating; she was just doing what she had to do to solve the task. She probably just experienced it as the everyday feeling we all have of sometimes changing our mind between two alternative courses of action.

If Dee could pull this kind of "trick" in the laboratory, then it seems likely that she was doing the same thing all the time in her everyday life. In fact, we got the impression—since she used the trick right from the start of the test session—that she had already learned, albeit unconsciously, that monitoring her own movements was a useful strategy. This kind of learning must have been happening almost as soon as Dee started to deal with her impoverished visual world. Such behavioral compensation is a natural way of dealing with the problems faced by any brain-damaged person: you do whatever you need to do to solve the problems that face you. You may not know how you are doing it, but if it works you adopt it. In fact, later on, Dee seems to have taken these behavioral aids a step further by internalizing the whole thing, so that she didn't even need to perform an action explicitly. She became able to cue herself just by *imagining* performing a particular action on the object in front of her, without actually doing it.

Our evidence for this internalization of Dee's self-monitoring strategy came from a study in which we asked her to show us the slant of a line drawn on a piece of paper by copying the line on a separate piece of paper. In theory she once more shouldn't have been able to do this: after all, it was just like asking her to match the orientation of a slot by rotating a card held in her hand. As we described early on in this book, she was quite unable to do that—at least, not at first. But we didn't mention then that it didn't take her long to learn a trick to deal with the slot-matching task—one that worked in much the same way as the self-correction ploy in the block-grasping task we have just described. What Dee did was to surreptitiously "break the rules" and move the card a little way toward the slot as if she were about to mail it, rather than holding it in place and just rotating it. Presumably she was partially engaging her visuomotor system by making this incipient posting movement. This way, she could line up the card with the orientation of the slot—and then hold it at that angle to offer her "perceptual report" of the slot. Again, it was not an attempt to cheat: like all of us, Dee wanted to do well, and this was how she could best solve the task she was given, which was to match the card to the orientation of the slot. In one sense it was a perfectly valid way of performing the task we gave her; it is just that the most natural way for most of us to do the task would be to use something Dee could not use: our visual experience of what the slot actually looks like.

So we should have guessed that Dee would adopt a similar sort of strategy, if she could, when asked to copy lines. And of course she did, at least until we told her not to. What she did was to "trace" a line in the air above each line we showed her, and then make the same movement on paper with the pencil. So her drawings were much more accurate than they should have been. But even when Dee agreed to stop tracing in the air, she continued to draw her lines far better than chance. In struggling to understand this, we noticed that her drawing movements still didn't look like normal copying. Dee would look fixedly at the original line for a few seconds each time, with her pencil on the other piece of paper, before then quickly drawing her line. Afterwards she confessed how she was doing it. Instead of explicitly tracing in the air over the top of the line, she *imagined* doing that, while keeping her pencil at the ready. She then drew her line quickly, before the imagined movement had faded from her mind. Since this ploy seemed to take Dee a few seconds, we thought that if we asked her to copy the line as soon as we presented it to her, she wouldn't have time to generate an imagined movement. The result was dramatic: Dee's lines were now drawn at random, and they showed no systematic relationship to the line she was shown. All she could now do was to guess. Only when she had time to imagine making a tracing movement was she able to draw a line that matched the original.

In all of these fascinating strategies, Dee was not so much telling us about what she could *see*, but rather about what she could *do*. In other words, she was using her intact visuomotor system in the dorsal stream, not to improve her *perception*, but rather as an *alternative* to perception, which allowed her to give the right answers to the problems we had presented her with. She was solving a problem that was designed to test perception without using perception at all.

There is a lesson here, which is recognized by all experienced clinicians who routinely test patients with brain damage. The fact that a patient passes a test doesn't mean that the patient is doing so in the way that the designer of the test intended. As the saying goes, "use whatever works." It is a natural and highly beneficial tendency of humans (and other animals) that if they cannot solve a problem in the most obvious way, they will try to solve it in other, less obvious, ways. This indeed is one of the major foundations of neurological rehabilitation: the therapist tries to find an alternative route by which the patient's deficits can be circumvented. Often these require specific training, but in many other cases, particularly over periods of years, patients will come up with effective strategies themselves. Dee is a good example of this.

To deal with everyday problems that would normally require perception of the form and shape of objects, Dee has to rely on strategies like those we have outlined here because her brain damage has completely devastated the ventral stream pathways that process form. As mentioned in Chapter 6, we have obtained objective confirmation of this ventral-stream damage from our brain imaging studies. Those studies, by providing both a confirmation and a clarification of what we had inferred on the basis of behavioral testing, illustrate the value of systematic neuropsychological investigations of patients with brain damage. In Dee's case, her pattern of impaired and intact visual abilities maps beautifully onto the patterns of brain activation in her ventral and dorsal streams as revealed by brain imaging. Taken together, the totality of our findings with Dee reflect not so much a recovery of damaged brain function, so much as her learning to exploit intact brain structures, in particular those in her dorsal stream. In this way, she is able to cope with the challenges facing her as she tries to live as full a life as possible within her diminished visual world. In short, her brain has adapted to the loss of one of its major components by a large-scale reorganization of how it controls itself. Rather like an ice hockey team that has lost a player because of penalties, the damaged brain has to adapt and form a new dynamic configuration. Like the team, if the brain does this, it can still perform well enough to cope successfully with the challenges it faces.

The story could have been very different if Dee had sustained her brain damage early in life, before puberty, while her brain was still developing and still retained a degree of plasticity. In such cases, the damage can often be bypassed, by co-opting pathways normally used by the brain for other purposes altogether. Unfortunately for Dee, she suffered her brain damage in adulthood. In contrast, another patient with visual form agnosia we have studied, Serge Blanc, suffered his very extensive brain damage as a result of a brain infection at age three. Serge's brain has recovered so much visual function that he is highly confident as he walks around new environments, and even rides a moped around the country lanes where he lives. He is also proficient at table tennis, swimming, and keeping goal in soccer—he can even catch two tennis balls at the same time, and juggle with them. Although he, like Dee, has enormous difficulties in recognizing shapes and patterns, he does have some conscious perception of the simple features of the pictures we show him. Sometimes he can painstakingly put these together and infer what it is he is looking at. Dee cannot do this. Functional imaging studies by Jean-François Démonet and Sandra Lê at Toulouse in France, suggest that Serge achieves this perception of simple lines and edges by redeploying parts of his parietal cortex as an alternative to his totally destroyed ventral stream.

Although the young developing brain has much greater ability to rewire itself than the mature brain, we now know that some limited rewiring can occur in the adult brain. The challenge is to work out how this happens and how it can be encouraged to happen even more. Introducing human stem cells (the developmental

203

precursors of all kinds of cells, including neurons) into damaged areas of the brain is one promising way ahead for scientists to explore how new brain circuits can be encouraged to replace the missing ones. Another promising avenue is the use of the brain's own chemicals to promote the growth of new connections and pathways in the human brain. Gene therapy is another possibility. Already, promising clinical trials are underway in which a number of retinal diseases, including color blindness, are being treated by injecting the genes for missing rods and cones into patients' eyes. Degenerative brain diseases, such as Parkinson's, are also being treated experimentally with targeted gene therapy. Similar treatments theoretically could be used to deal with damage to the brain, to regrow neural tissue that is specific to the damaged region. All of this lies in the future, but there is real scope for optimism that within a few years the kinds of brain damage we have seen in Dee would not be irreversible, and that people like her could once again come to see the world with the full richness that the rest of us normally take for granted.

Summary

Although Dee has learned to cope with her visual disabilities remarkably well, careful behavioral testing reveals that her damaged perceptual system has shown little true recovery in the more than twenty years since her accident. She has learned to use visuomotor tricks to compensate for the absence of form perception, but her object recognition deficits are still apparent when we take care to prevent her from using these various coping strategies. Our anatomical and functional magnetic resonance images of her brain have provided powerful confirmation of the conclusions we drew from our earlier behavioral work with Dee. In fact, the neuroimaging evidence could not be more clear: Dee's ventral stream is severely damaged, but her dorsal stream appears to be working relatively normally. However, the functional neuroimaging evidence is also giving us new information that goes well beyond our earlier speculations. For example, we are finding significant activation of certain areas within the ventral stream that have *not* been lost—presumably either because information is getting through along essentially normal routes, or because new routes have opened up. Further investigation of these patterns of activation, and how they change when Dee views different pictures and scenes, promise to reveal new insights into the ventral stream's normal modus operandi, as well as information about the brain areas that are called into service when she engages in new strategies to get around her impairments. The remarkable visuomotor adaptations that Dee has acquired over the years provide a powerful testimony to the robustness of the human condition. Studying the way the brain reorganizes itself in response to severe damage presents one of the most important challenges to neuroscience in the 21st century.

Further Reading

Our discoveries of some of Dee's strategies for dealing with perceptual tasks are detailed in these two articles:

Dijkerman, H.C. and Milner, A.D. (1997). Copying without perceiving: motor imagery in visual form agnosia. *Neuroreport, 8,*729–732.

Murphy, K.J., Racicot, C.I., and Goodale, M.A. (1996). The use of visuomotor cues as a strategy for making perceptual judgments in a patient with visual form agnosia. *Neuropsychology, 10,* 396–401.

This paper provides a description of "Serge Blanc," the second patient with visual form agnosia we have been able to study in some detail, and who differs from Dee in having had almost all of his life to adjust to his visual deficits:

Lê, S., Cardebat, D., Boulanouar, K., Hénaff, M.A., Michel, F., Milner, A.D., Dijkerman, H.C., Puel, M., and Démonet, J.F. (2002). Seeing, since childhood, without ventral stream: a behavioural study. *Brain, 125,* 58–74.

For accessible accounts of how experience can shape our brain—and how experience can be manipulated to rehabilitate individuals with brain damage—see these two books:

Doidge, N. (2007). *The Brain that Changes Itself: Stories of personal triumph from the frontiers of brain science.* London: Penguin.

Robertson, I.H. (1999): *Mind Sculpture: Unlocking your brain's untapped potential.* New York, NY: Fromm International.

For more detailed information on this topic, readers may wish to consult this book containing contributions from numerous experts in the field:

Raskin, S. (2011). *Neuroplasticity and Neurorehabilitation.* New York, NY: Guilford Press.

INDEX